Labor and Birth

Labor and Birth

A Coaching Guide for Fathers and Friends

Cecilia Worth

Introduction by Elisabeth Bing

Illustrations by Judith MacLaughlin and Kathleen F. Anderson

McGraw-Hill Book Company

New York St. Louis San Francisco Bogotá Guatemala Hamburg Lisbon
Madrid Mexico Montreal Panama Paris San Juan São Paulo Tokyo Toronto

Copyright © 1983 by Cecilia Worth

All rights reserved. Printed in the United States of America. Except as permitted under the Copyright Act of 1976, no part of this publication may be reproduced or distributed in any form or by any means, or stored in a data base or retrieval system, without the prior written permission of the publisher.

123456789 DOC DOC 876543

ISBN 0-07-071817-2{PBK.}
ISBN 0-07-071818-0{H.C.}

LIBRARY OF CONGRESS CATALOGING IN PUBLICATION DATA

Worth, Cecilia.
Labor and birth.
(Having a baby / by Cecilia Worth)
1. Labor (Obstetrics) I. Title.
II. Series: Worth,
Cecilia. Having a baby.
RG652.W66   1983   618'.4   82-13029
ISBN 0-07-071818-0
ISBN 0-07-071817-2 (pbk.)

A Sun Words book
Edited by Sandra Oddo

*Written in recognition
of all those who are dedicated
to serving expectant parents
with respect, intelligence, and love.*

*Dedicated, with love,
to all my students
throughout the years
who have shared their experiences with me
so that future parents can benefit
from information that can come only
from on-the-spot accounts.*

Foreword

The childbearing years are among the most dramatic and exciting periods of anybody's life.

Most of us these days do not grow up in extended families, where it would be a matter of growing up to learn about childbirth, nursing, parenting. Now, we might learn in school all the scientific facts about birthing, but this knowledge comes to us at an age when we are not particularly interested in the facts or the psychological impacts of birthing and parenting. We can't identify yet; there are too many other things we have to do first, before we consider childbearing.

However, for most of us the time comes when it seems imperative that we find answers to our questions. We need knowledge and facts to replace our fantasies about childbirth. It is an exhilarating time, and for many of us it means finding out, reading, asking questions.

Cecilia Worth's book series will answer just about everything we would want to know. Cecilia and I have been friends for many, many years. I have always admired the author's active mind, her questioning, her interest and her utter humanity when dealing with others, and in particular with her childbirth students. Her book series shows what kind of woman she is: precise, to the point, and full of understanding. In her series she talks to all people who are at a time of their lives when they need her advice and wisdom.

The special attraction of Cecilia's books is that they are short, accurate, easy to read, and still full of an enormous amount of information. They are written for the very busy professional woman as well as for the woman who finds it difficult to get answers in a more extensive book. They are written for the very young mother and father as well as for the older ones. They are books that answer the many questions of the dark and grey areas we all experience when it comes to childbearing.

I know that it is not easy to confine one's writing to essentials, but that is exactly what the author has done. Her books are full of facts, full of practical knowledge, and they are written in an easy and relaxed way, as if the author were talking personally to each of us.

Elisabeth Bing

Contents

Foreword   vii

Letter to a Labor Coach   1

1. What Coaching Means   5

2. What Is Labor Like?   11

3. The Mother's Skills for Working with Labor   21
   Relaxing   25
   Breathing   29
   Pushing   43
   Positions for Birth   53
   The Importance of Practicing   59
   Quick Guide to Mother's Labor Skills   62

4. Waiting for Labor to Start   67

5. Going to the Hospital   87

6. The Coach's Skills (General Principles)   101
   Quick Coaching Guide (General Principles)   123

7. The Coach's Skills (Stages of Labor)   127
    Quick Coaching Guide (Early & Active Labor)   162
    Quick Coaching Guide (Transition)   163
    Quick Coaching Guide (Pushing)   164
    Quick Coaching Guide (Birth)   166

8. The Coach's Skills (After the Birth)   169
    Quick Coaching Guide (After the Birth)   184

9. Coping with Pain   187
    Quick Coaching Guide (Regaining Control)   191

10. Born on the Way to the Hospital   193

11. What to Expect with Hospital and Medical Procedures   205
    Undressing   205
    Vital Signs   206
    Urinalysis   206
    Internal Exams   206
    Patient's History   207
    Blood Tests   209
    Shave   209
    Enema   210
    IVs   212
    Fetal Monitor   213

Rupturing the Membrane   216
Episiotomy   217
Silver Nitrate Medication   219
Circumcision   220
Medication   221

12. What to Expect with Variations in Labor   235
    Hyperventilation   235
    Forceps   238
    X-Rays   241
    Back Labor   244
    Induced and Supplemented Labor   250
    Cesarean Birth   252

13. Loss: Prematurity, a Less-than-Perfect Baby, Death   275

14. Lists   287
    Questions to Ask the Hospital in Advance   287
    Questions to Ask Midwife or Doctor   292
    Items to Bring from Home for Labor   295

15. Further Reading   299

16. Glossary   302

Letter to a Labor Coach

A labor coach is often the father of the baby soon to be born. Sometimes a caring relative or close friend of the expectant mother may volunteer for this exciting role. Whether you volunteered or were asked to be a coach, you may be wondering:

- How will I know what to do when?
- Will I be able to take it?
- How will I know which jobs are mine and which are the midwife's, the doctor's, or the nurse's?
- Will I remember everything?
- How will I act when the baby is born?

    This book is written to show you how to help someone through labor step by step. It describes coaching techniques that have proved effective in thousands of labors.

    These techniques are surprisingly simple. All you need are some basic facts, some skills acquired through practice, and a large supply of energy, patience, and love.

    The book will be most useful if you know its contents well. There is a great deal of information here. You need not try to memorize it; just read it carefully many times. You will see bullets (like this: •)

wherever there is a specific action you can take as a coach. As you read, underline or put a check mark next to the parts you especially want to remember. Then, when you need information quickly, you will know where to look for it.

- As you read, add your own notes.
- Use the suggestions when you and your partner practice together.

The guide is written to be easy to follow. Chapters are arranged to give you information in roughly the order you will need it—first, the physical process of labor and birth, and the skills a mother needs to work with her body; then, how to recognize labor when it starts and what to expect as you go to the hospital; after that, the skills you will need as labor coach. Next, there are chapters on variations in labor and on medical procedures, to prepare you for the unexpected, should it occur.

The information is concise. You can tuck the book into your pocket when labor begins and carry it with you to the hospital. During labor, when you need reminders they will be close at hand.

When people talk about their own labors and births, they often eloquently express the essence behind the facts and practical suggestions presented at much greater length by an author or teacher. The personal experiences presented in italic type throughout this book, related by people who have been my students over the years, bring the text to life. Better than anything else could, the variety of opinions, feelings, and experiences prove how every labor and birth, while following a basic pattern, is different for every individual.

Reading this book may be a little like rehearsing a play. You get to know the roles and the setting before the show goes on. But just as a performance is different from a rehearsal, using a technique in labor is very different from learning it in class and practicing it at home. So *Labor and Birth* is a kind of script that reviews the facts of childbirth and the techniques you and your partner will use.

This book is not a substitute for the classes that teach you and your partner these techniques. There is nothing like person-to-person learning. Classes usually will give you pointers about the hospitals you will use, too. And sometimes hospitals require classes before a mother may have a helper with her during labor and birth.

Throughout this book, the mother is called the partner of her coach rather than the wife. For one thing, the coach may be a friend or relative rather than the husband. For another, the term "wife" is inaccurate for the many couples who choose not to marry. More important, however, working together during labor *is* a partnership, a profound sharing of the effort, fortitude, and love that create the teamwork to bring about the miracle of giving birth.

You have my sincere wishes for an enriching and rewarding experience.

Cecilia Worth

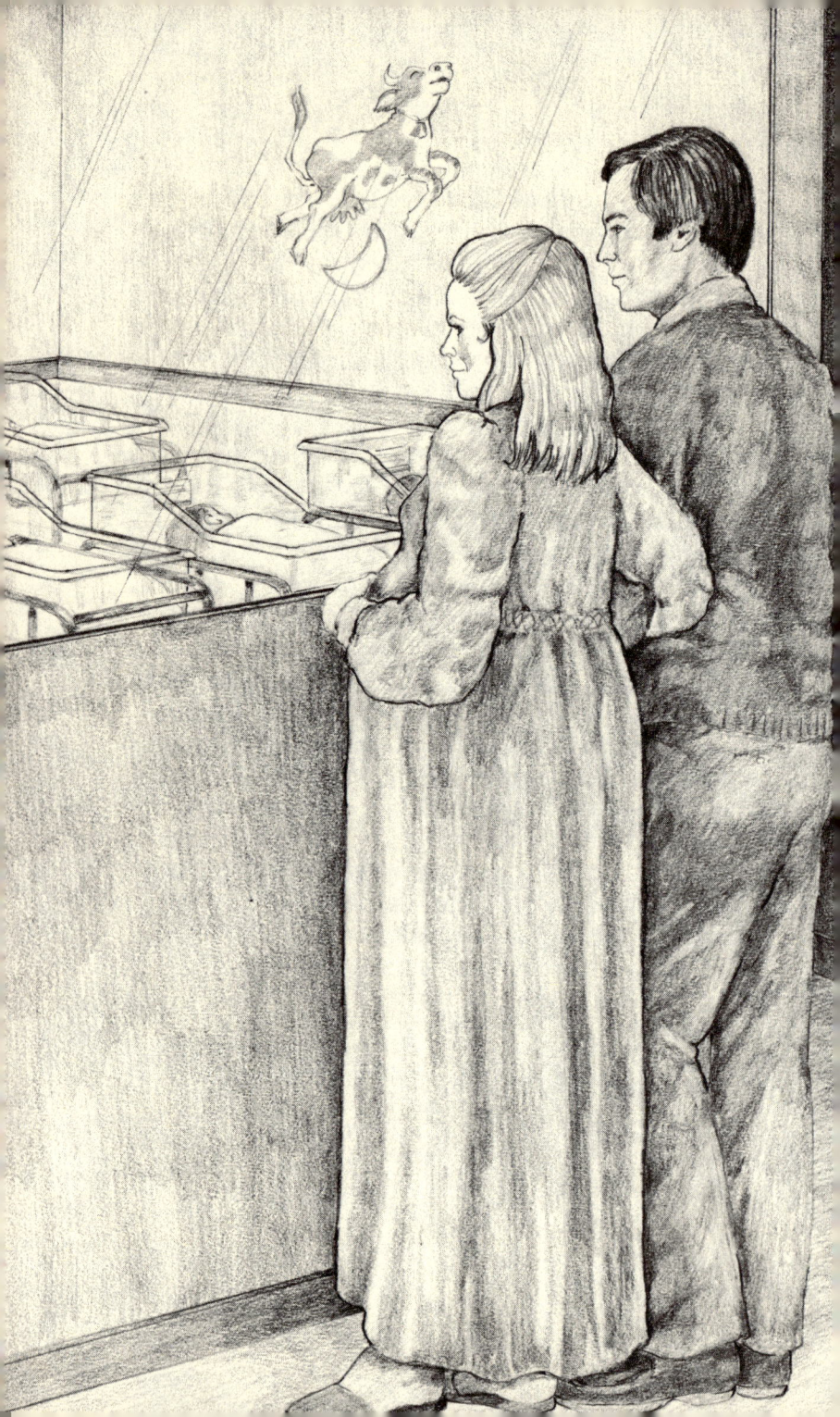

1. What Coaching Means

Helping a woman through labor and being present at the birth of a baby can be one of the most satisfying, rewarding, and amazing experiences of a lifetime.

Coaching is not difficult, though it can be tiring, frustrating, and demanding. It does not require years of knowledge and know-how, though it does require special skills. A well-prepared coach knows a few basic techniques well, and uses them over and over. How you use those techniques is almost as important as knowing what they are.

Labor, just as its name suggests, is hard work. For expectant mothers, the idea of being in labor can be frightening. Women are concerned about the baby's well-being and their own. They worry about pain and wonder how they will manage contractions that hurt. There are two sides to the experience of a woman who is giving birth. On one side is the desire to stay in control and cope, using the skills she has learned. On the other side is the temptation to give in to fear and pain. Throughout the labor the balance goes back and forth between the two sides. The trick is to keep the scales tipped in favor of working *with* the experience. The more challenging the labor, the harder the effort.

A lot depends on how well a woman knows and can use her techniques. Her physical condition is also important. So is the kind of labor, the quality of her surroundings—and, most important, the kind of support she has (or doesn't have).

All the people with whom she has contact influence a woman's feelings during labor. Someone who cares about her, who will keep her steady company and guide and encourage her, tips the balance in her favor.

This is where you come in.

□ □ □

"At the beginning we talked, held hands, and just smiled between contractions and his presence was reassuring. As the contractions grew stronger, his presence was a psychological necessity and I could never have continued without him."

"They all made me feel that Karen's birth was the only thing in the universe that had any importance that day."

□ □ □

First, you must know your partner's skills. Basically, these are

Relaxing

Breathing

Pushing

These skills are reviewed in the chapter on *The Mother's Skills for Working with Labor*, which starts on page 21.

If you have tried these yourself, you can guide your partner when she needs help in using them. You must know them well enough to spot errors and to offer reminders.

"When I tried relaxing at the dentist's, I discovered how easily my shoulders tensed up. So I knew to keep a close watch there during Mary's contractions."

□ □ □

Second, you must know your own coaching skills. In labor, your partner is the star; you are the director. *The Coach's Skills,* which starts on page 101, explains ways to:

1. Give your partner confidence.
2. Calm her.
3. Keep her going when she is tired.
4. Make her comfortable.
5. Help her to stay in control.
6. Act as her advocate and interpreter with the other people around her.
7. Help her to use her techniques in the best way she can under circumstances that may be unfamiliar, or may change.

□ □ □

"A gentle touch, a head wiped with a cool cloth are better than a hundred sour lollipops."

□ □ □

Third, understanding is important. The better you understand what is going on, both with the process of labor and with the routines and practices of hospitals and medical attendants, the more confident you will be in using your techniques when and where they will help the most. These points are outlined in *What Is*

Labor Like? (page 11), *What to Expect with Hospital and Medical Procedures* (page 205), and *What to Expect with Variations in Labor* (page 235).

Fourth, you should be prepared to help yourself. You must deal with the concerns or worries common to many coaches-to-be. Will you faint? Get sick? Find it impossible to tolerate seeing your partner in pain? Usually these concerns are not a problem when you are prepared. You can concentrate on helping, rather than putting time and energy into trying to figure out what is going on. The more you know, the more involved you get. You are a participant rather than an onlooker, and too busy and too interested to feel ill. You are part of the team that is working to bring this baby into the world safely.

To be prepared, both for your partner and for yourself, get all the exposure you can, in addition to reading this book. For prepared childbirth, training is essential unless you and your partner are lucky enough to have a nurse who can stay with you throughout labor, instruct you both step by step, and still make time for her nursing duties.

Training is usually given either privately or in hospitals. In addition, take a tour of your hospital (or hospitals, if your midwife or doctor works at more than one). Explore *all* the birth settings available to you, including birthing rooms in hospitals, and independent birthing centers.

With your partner or by yourself, meet and talk often with your midwife or doctor (and, if yours belongs to a group practice, meet with the other members of the practice). Share your views. Explain your requests. Learn theirs. In this way, you all get to know each other a little, and you start to form the team of which you will be a part during the labor and birth (and, if you cannot agree on important points no matter how hard you try, you will still have time to consider going elsewhere).

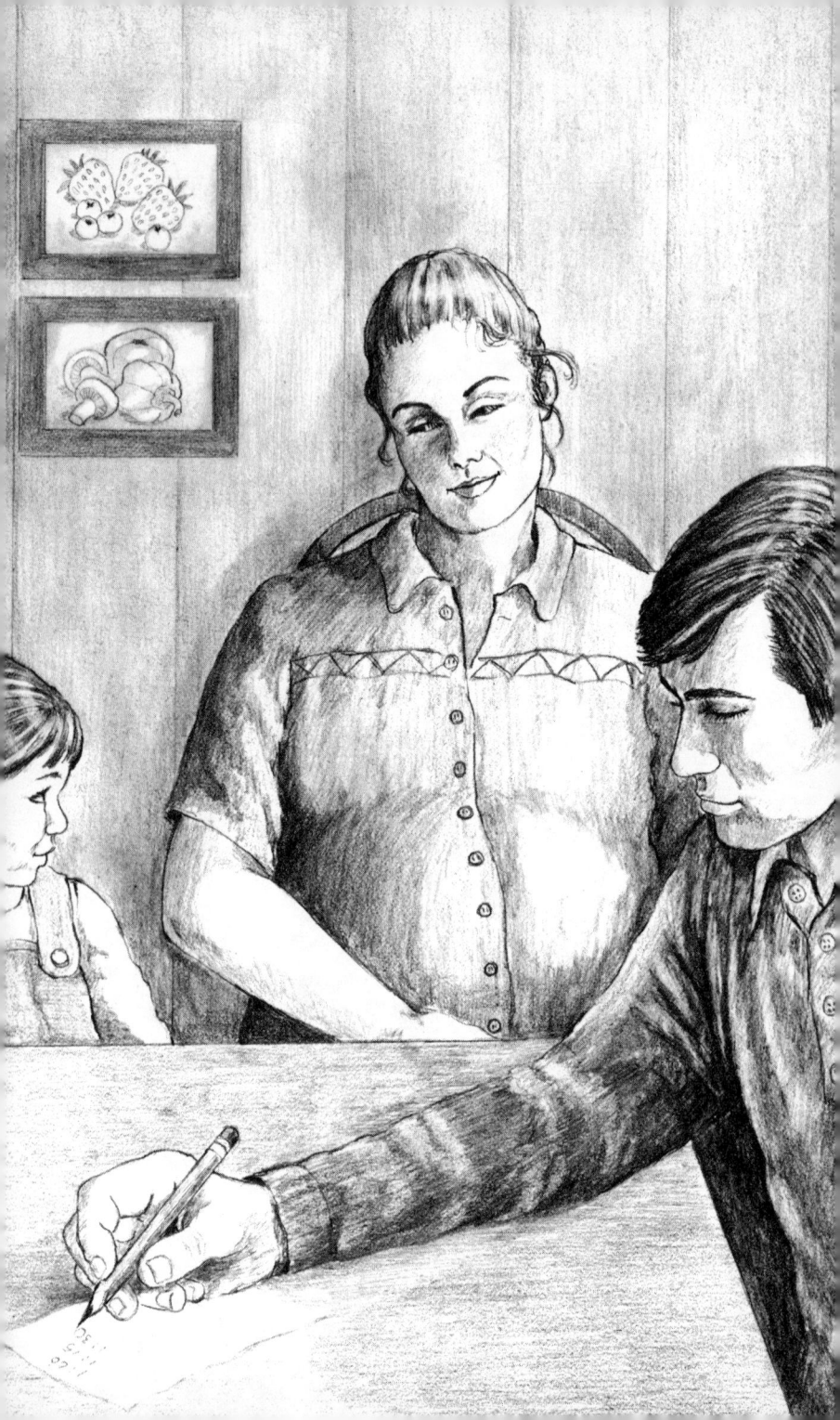

2. What Is Labor Like?

Women and men alike wonder about coping with something they have never experienced or perhaps have experienced with difficulty. Usually we put together our own pictures of what will happen, based on a few facts and a lot of imagination. But what will the real thing be like?

The labor described in the next chapters is an *average* picture put together from the labors of thousands of women. Textbook labors like this, however, are rare. For each woman, whether she is a first-time mother or a mother with several children, each labor is highly individual. Each has its share of surprises. For example, the way labor begins may be different from what you had expected. Contractions may feel different to your partner from the way she had imagined them. You may be surprised by a short or a long labor, or by back labor (page 244), or an induced labor (page 250), or even a Cesarean (page 252).

Often we react to the unexpected as if something were going wrong. We become frightened and rattled and tense. Thinking gets foggy. But most variations are normal, and if you need to make certain, get the facts. Never hesitate to phone your midwife or doctor at any time of day or night when you are at home. In the hospital, speak to your labor nurse or ask her to get your midwife or doctor for you. If she or he is out of the hospital, you can always call from a hospital pay phone. Being reassured is a necessity, if you and

Inside the uterus

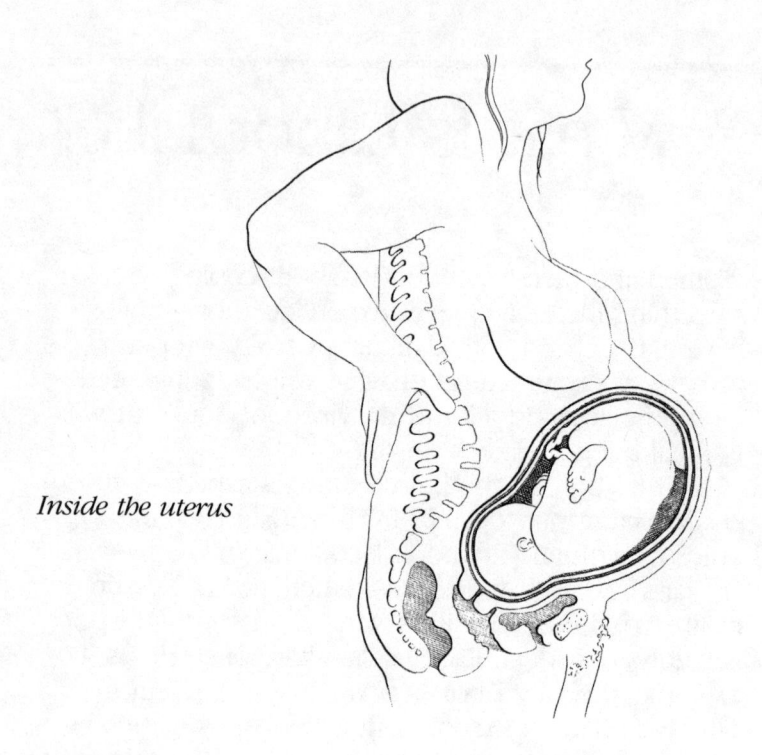

your partner are to work with, instead of against, yourselves during labor.

INSIDE THE UTERUS

The uterus is shaped like an upside-down balloon with its opening underneath. This opening to the uterus, the cervix, is long and fat, like the neck of a turtleneck sweater. A baby, ready to be born, can fit through this opening because it stretches and widens, very much like a turtleneck sweater stretching and widening to fit over someone's head.

The uterus is made of muscle fibres. All through

pregnancy these fibres tighten (contract) and relax. In early pregnancy the fibres contract independently of one another. Later in pregnancy they contract in little groups. In labor they all work together as a unit. They are like members of a team in training who work out on their own until the big event.

These non-labor contractions, called **Braxton-Hicks contractions**, usually are not felt by the mother until the seventh month or so. They are mild or moderate in strength. Labor contractions are much stronger because they must open the uterus and move the baby out into the world.

During the last month of pregnancy, especially for a first-time mother, the uterus prepares by flattening (effacing) the cervix almost completely (95 percent). The cervix begins to open (dilate) by as much as 4 of the total width of 10 centimeters, or 2 of the total width of 5 fingers.

During labor, the muscle fibres work together, contracting and relaxing until the uterus has stretched the cervix open, pushed the baby out into the world, and passed the afterbirth (the placenta that nourished the baby before birth, the water bag that protected it, and the remainder of the umbilical cord).

Labor contractions repeat a pattern, working and resting, working and resting, over and over. Usually the labor contractions start slowly and gently. The uterus contracts for about 30 seconds, then rests for somewhere between 5 and 20 minutes. Though this pattern usually leads to more active labor after a few hours, it may start and stop over a period of several days. If a woman has a vaginal exam during this period she may be disappointed to discover that her cervix has not opened much more than it was at her last routine office visit.

STAGES OF LABOR

Labor itself is divided into 3 parts, called stages: flattening and opening of the cervix, birth, and afterbirth.

The first stage is also divided into 3 parts or phases: early labor or warm-up, active labor, and transition.

FIRST STAGE: EARLY LABOR

These hours of early labor are a warm-up time. Usually there is little progress.

Average total time: 8 to 9 hours with a first baby, or half this time with subsequent babies. These times vary tremendously from one woman to another, and from one labor to another.

Slow progress: The cervix can efface up to 95 percent, and dilate up to 3 centimeters, or 1½ fingers (but that much progress is not guaranteed).

Contractions last 30 to 60 seconds, with mild to moderate strength that may vary from one contraction to another.

Intervals last longer than 5 minutes (first baby) or longer than 8 minutes (later babies).

Pattern of contractions is usually regular, although it may be uneven.

Mother's feelings may be excited, nervous, energetic, calm.

FIRST STAGE: ACTIVE LABOR

Progress begins, with big changes in the cervix.

Average total time: 3 to 6 hours (first baby); 1 to 2 hours (subsequent babies). Remember that these times vary from labor to labor.

Cervix effaces more than during early labor (up to 95 percent possible); and dilates to 6 or 7 centimeters, or 3 to 3½ fingers.

Contractions last 45 to 60 seconds, and are moderate or strong. They may become stronger gradually over a period of hours or quickly, within minutes.

Intervals last 5 minutes or less (first baby); 8 minutes or less (later babies).

Pattern of contractions is usually regular although it may not be, especially with back labor (see page 248).

Mother's feelings may be serious, thoughtful, nervous, calm, frightened, quiet, very sensitive, self-involved.

FIRST STAGE: TRANSITION

This is the final dilation of the cervix before the second stage starts.

Average total time: 5 minutes to 2 hours (first babies usually take the longest time).

Cervix becomes fully effaced and fully dilated, at 10 centimeters or a width of 5 fingers.

Contractions average 60 to 90 seconds, and are strong.

Intervals average 30 to 60 seconds, and at times are missing entirely.

Pattern of contractions is usually regular.

Mother's feelings may be restless, short-tempered,

Contractions: First Stage of Labor

30 seconds

20 minutes to 5 minutes

Early Labor (Warm-Up)

60 seconds

5 minutes to 2 minutes

Active Labor

90 to 60 seconds

1 minute to ½ minute

Contractions: Second Stage of Labor

Transition

60 seconds

3 minutes to 2 minutes

Contractions: Third Stage of Labor

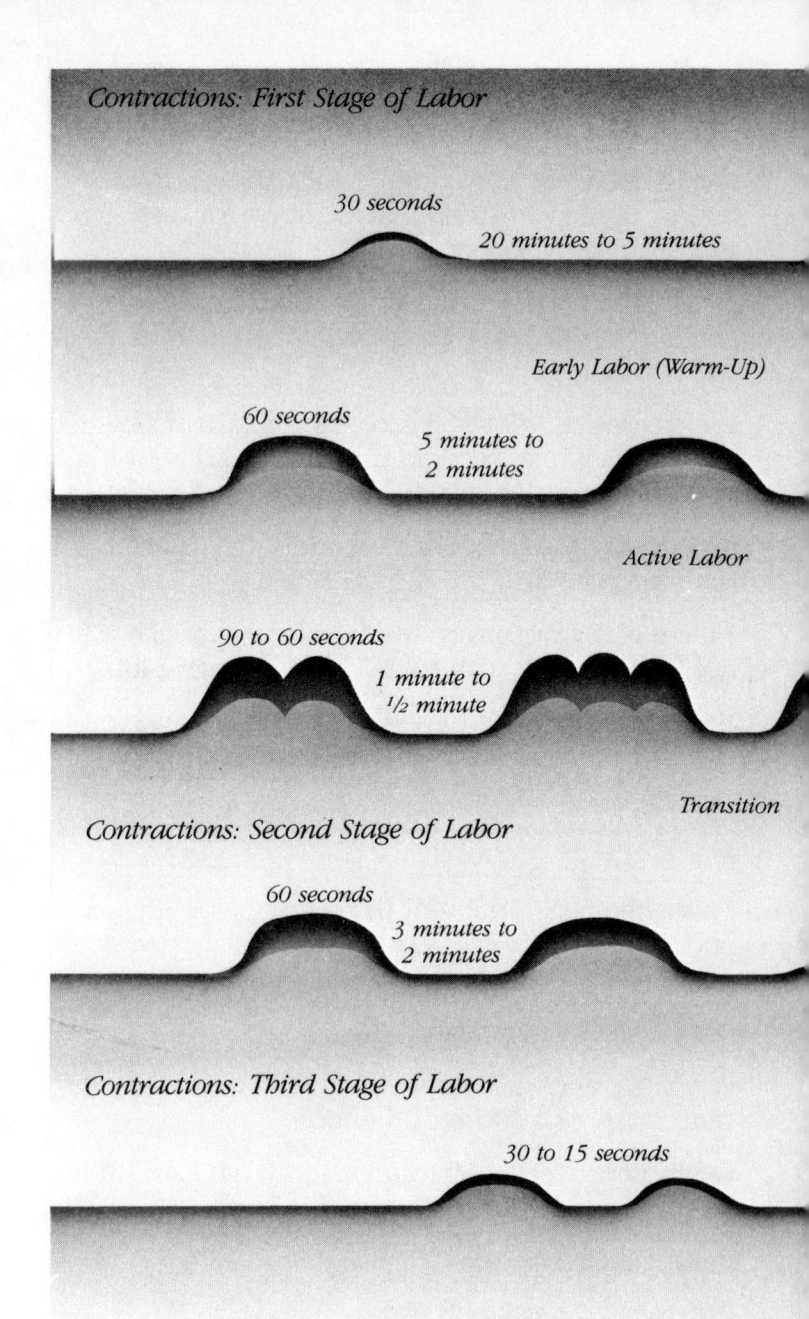

30 to 15 seconds

Pattern of contractions in an average labor. The shading of ea

Miniature rest periods in mid-contraction

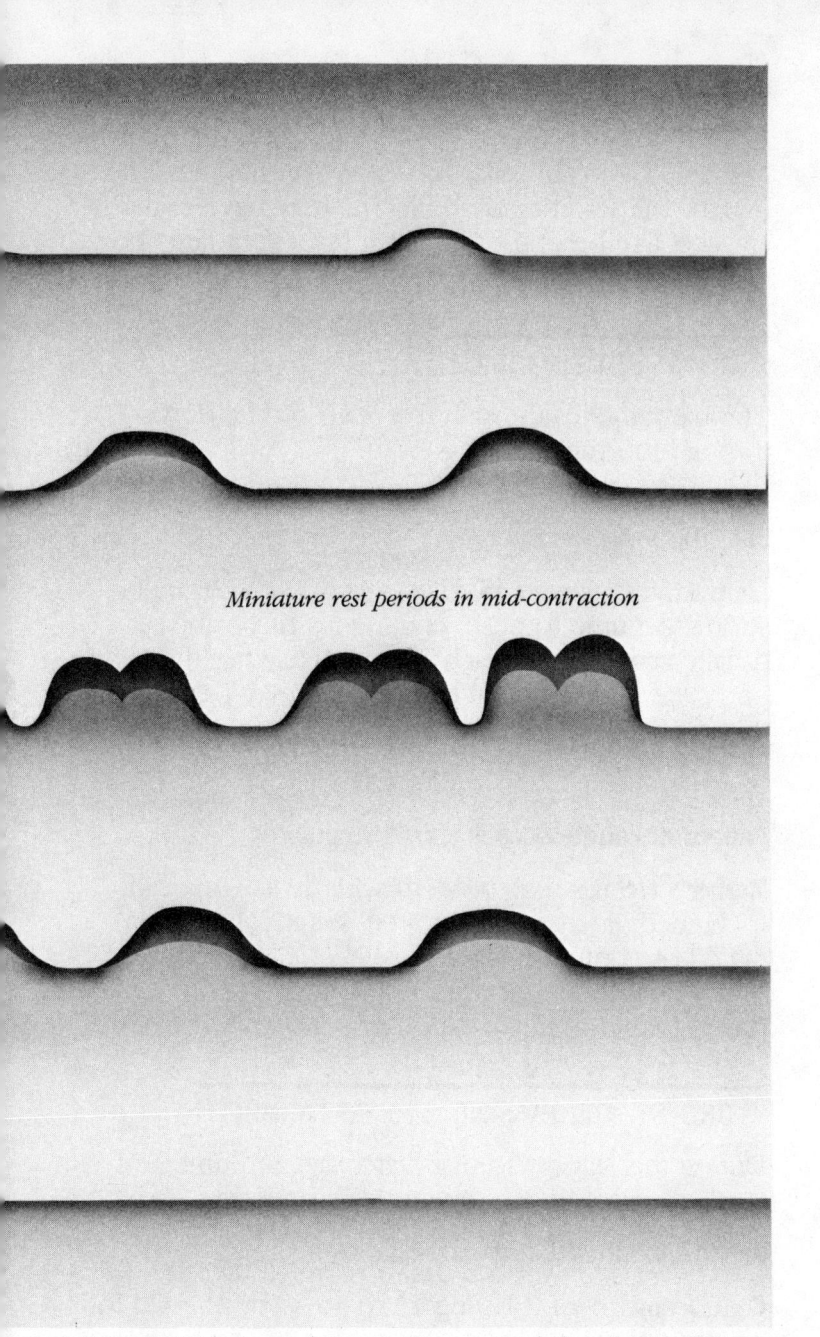

ontraction shows how each grows more—and then less—strong.

frightened, discouraged, very sensitive, trapped. She may be nauseated and vomit. She may have backache and feel like bearing down (as if for a very large bowel movement) during contractions.

SECOND STAGE: BIRTH

The baby moves through the open cervix, down through the vagina, and is born.

Average total time: 5 minutes to 2 hours (first babies take the longer time).

Contractions average 45 to 60 seconds, moderate or strong. An urge to push, continuous or on-and-off, usually accompanies each contraction. After the second stage starts, several contractions may pass before this urge comes on.

Intervals average 2 to 4 minutes.

Pattern of contractions is usually regular.

Mother's feelings may be alert, wide-awake, excited, frightened, energetic, very tired, self-involved, calm, rattled or confused. She usually feels like bearing down during contractions, either intermittently or constantly, either mildly or strongly.

THIRD STAGE: PASSING THE AFTERBIRTH

During this stage placenta, water sac, and umbilical cord are passed from the mother's body.

Average total time: 5 to 30 minutes.

Contractions: 1 or 2 lasting 15 to 30 seconds, mild to moderate.

Mother's feelings may be very happy, dazed, energized, very tired, physically very sensitive.

> **Watch for sudden progress spurts**, sometimes with a first baby, *often* with others.

Note: All these estimates of time are flexible. An *average* labor is described, put together from the experiences of thousands of mothers. Relying on facts is always more reassuring than juggling possibilities—but each labor is different from every other, even for someone who has had many babies. "Facts" in labor have many variations. Most variations in labor are normal and to be expected. Those variations made up the averages in the first place.

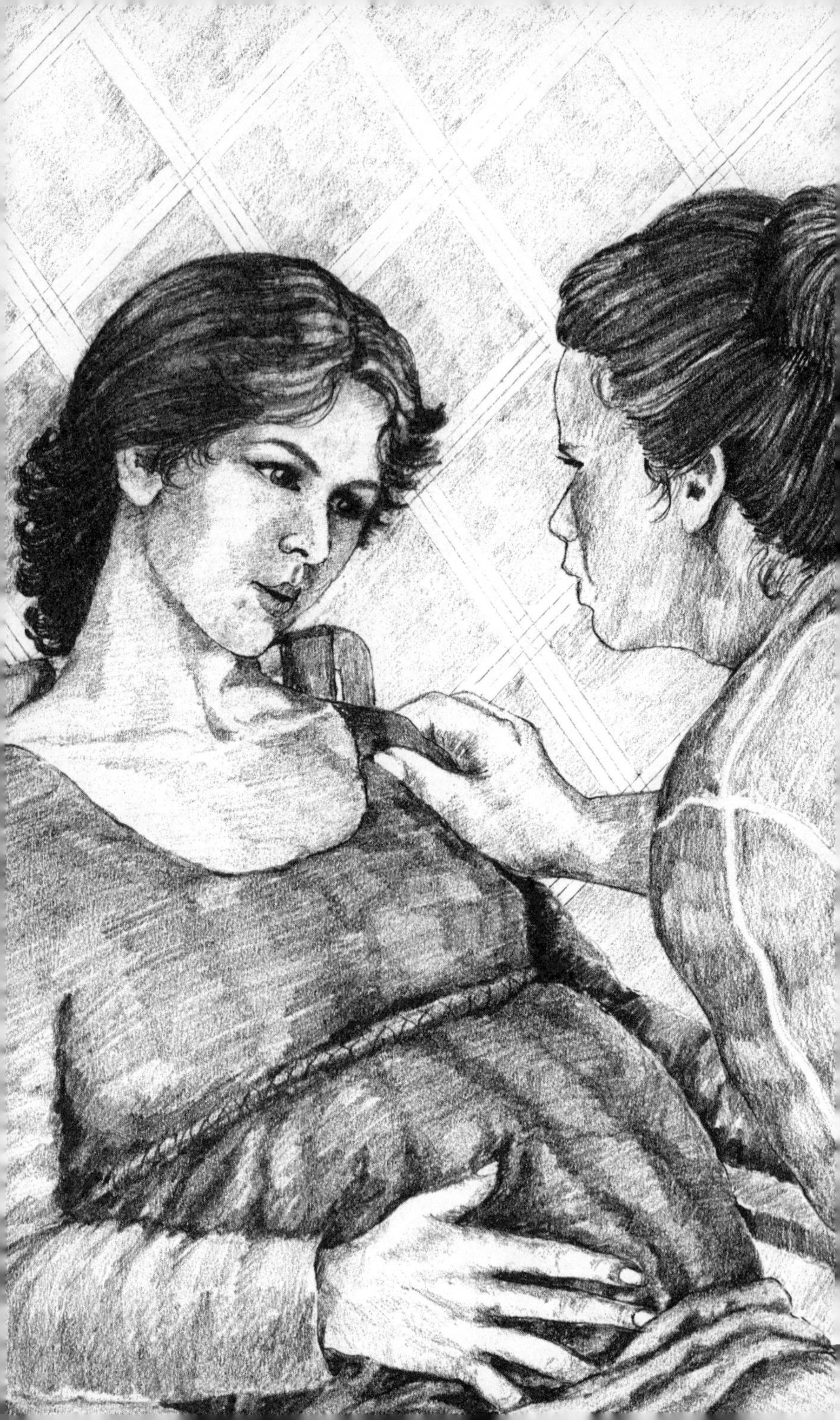

3. The Mother's Skills for Working with Labor

The skills a mother uses in labor are taught and written about a little differently by everyone. Some techniques are grouped together under special names—the Lamaze method, the Bradley method, the Read method—but all share similar goals. A mother who knows how to relax, breathe, and push can feel that she has some influence over what is happening instead of being controlled by the forces of labor. She can work with her body instead of against it. Pain becomes something she can face and cope with instead of something that makes her feel overwhelmed and helpless.

To make coaching work, you must learn your partner's labor skills. First, you cannot fully understand her skills if you have never practiced them yourself. You have to be able to experience them as well as understand them. A baseball coach cannot guide a player if he himself has never swung a bat. He will not play in the game, just as you will not have the contractions, but he does know how.

Second, during labor you may have to do these techniques with your partner. A painful contraction can make her lose control. A moment of nervousness can confuse her. Being tired can cause her to forget.

Spoken instructions sometimes hinder instead of help because she has to figure out how to follow them. When she is under pressure, thinking clearly is difficult. At these times, actions speak louder than words. Copying your demonstration is the quickest and easiest way for your partner to get back on the track.

A mother has 3 basic tools for handling labor:

Relaxing

Breathing

Pushing

all held together by **concentration.** The **cleansing breath**, and **focus** help her to center her energy.

CONCENTRATION

Concentration is one key to working with labor. When a woman's body is actively at work, as it is in labor, she naturally responds with a great outpouring of energy. She wants to *do* something. This energy can be scattered and drained away when a woman tenses up and struggles against what she is feeling. Instead, she can gather her energy and concentrate it on helpful ways to respond to her labor. She must think steadily about what she is doing and not allow distractions such as pain, fear, or noise to turn her attention elsewhere. Whenever your partner is trying to cope, and during contractions especially, concentration can help her to calm herself and to stay in control.

□ □ □

"The more I concentrated on how I was breathing, the more I could ride with how the contractions were feeling."

THE CLEANSING BREATH

This is a long, slow breath that begins and ends every contraction. It is carefully rehearsed so that, long before actual labor, it becomes an unconscious signal to start and stop working. Doing it when a contraction begins says "Gather your forces and face the contraction. Concentrate. Give it all your attention." Doing it when a contraction ends says "Let go of the contraction completely. Think only of resting." Without the cleansing breath at the beginning, a woman meets her contraction feeling half-ready. Without the breath at the end, she tends to hold onto the memory of the last contraction, waiting tensely for the next.

The quick switch of attention from working to resting is especially important when contractions are long and strong, and intervals are very short. Even 30 seconds of complete rest can supply energy for the next contraction.

The **cleansing breath** is taken in through the nose and blown out through the mouth, slowly and easily to set the pace for working with the contraction itself.

To practice:
Have your partner use a cleansing breath to start and end every exercise.

FOCUS

Focusing is a technique to help maintain concentration. A woman rests her eyes on a particular object or area while she concentrates. Shutting her eyes tends to cause her to focus on inner fear and pain. She needs her eyes open to keep her in touch with reality—her coach and her surroundings—without being distracted by looking around at them.

□ □ □

"He kept nagging me to keep my eyes open, but I found it easier to squint sort of, and look at but not really see what I was staring at—like spacing out when you're meditating. I used a doorknob or the labor room sign."

□ □ □

Eyes should rest lightly on an object—**the focal point**—without staring intensely, almost without seeing it. This prevents eye fatigue.

To practice:
Have your partner use a focal point while practicing every exercise. She will get into the habit of using it as she does cleansing breaths, so that it will be more automatic during contractions.

At times, when strong contractions interfere with your partner's concentration, she can focus on your face as you guide her through relaxing and breathing.

□ □ □

"I used my husband's eyes and a scar he has on his top lip as focal points."

□ □ □

RELAXING

Relaxing is the other key to working with labor. It is used:

1. By itself with contractions.

2. As a foundation for all the breathing skills.

3. To help the mother to cope with physical or emotional discomfort.

Consider what relaxing can do: It saves energy. Tension uses energy. Tightened muscles are at work using oxygen and nutrients meant for other body functions. In labor, tension uses some of the fuel meant for the uterus. It steals energy from the mother, lessening her stamina and tiring her. Both the mother and her uterus need all the energy they can get. Without that energy, progress is slow. Letting go of tension helps the uterus and mother to work at top level.

Relaxing is calming. When you are nervous, angry, or unhappy, with your mind rattling along full of questions and thoughts, consciously letting go of physical tension slows you down and soothes you. You may still have the worries, but they clamour less loudly and you feel more in control.

Relaxing in labor is different from the kind of relaxing you might do at the end of a long, hard day. A mother cannot simply slip into it. It is a definite skill and, in its way, a kind of work. It calls for a conscious effort to loosen one body part after another, over and over. She must pay constant attention to all the parts of herself where tension comes sneaking back. To do this during a contraction requires enormous concentration and constant reminders.

HEAD-TO-TOE RELEASING

Here is a very good routine for learning how to relax. It is followed by a special technique called *4-point releasing* for use during labor. Try them both yourself, then show them to your partner. If you and she already are familiar with relaxing skills, these may give you additional valuable pointers. The techniques are simple, and with the constant practice you should do, they will become a dependable response to stress—during labor and at other times as well.

Choose a location for practice that is private and quiet. Later, when you have learned the basics, choose a variety of places to practice. Surroundings during labor may be busy and noisy, so it is realistic to learn to release tension in a variety of circumstances.

Try giving directions like these to your partner as she practices and when she is in labor: "Let every single body part go limp, one at a time. Start with your forehead, and go all the way down to your toes. Leave nothing out, including the muscles between your legs (the perineum). Let go with one body part before you move on to another."

When you work with your partner, speak the name of every body part and, when it is possible, touch each one as you go. Lift an arm, a hand. Is it floppy or stiff? Does it drop when you let go or hold itself up? Relaxed muscles are soft. Tense muscles are hard. Have your partner tell you which body parts are hardest for her to loosen. Rest the flat of your hand against a tense spot. Tell her to let the warmth of your hand soak up the tension. Stroke her back, shoulders, each arm and leg, with your hand going in one direction, as though you are gently pulling the tension down and out of her body. Take all the time you need, using at least least 3 to 5 minutes.

Speak quietly. Tell her to *concentrate* on letting go, one body part at a time. It may be best to avoid the word "relax" because sometimes it has the opposite effect. Use words that say exactly what you want her to do: "Release, let go, loosen, feel limp, heavy, drop your shoulders, loosen your body, release your hands, let go with your bottom (perineum)."

In addition to practicing during the day, have your partner do head-to-toe relaxing every night in bed before she goes to sleep. She will develop the habit of falling asleep afterward, and may be able to do the same in early labor, even though she is nervous or excited.

Notice that other nearby body parts let go out of habit, gained from the head-to-toe releasing. Practice 4-point releasing by itself, as it will be used in labor. Also practice it following head-to-toe releasing, as a reminder to *all* body parts to let go, too.

4-Point Releasing can produce the same result as head-to-toe releasing, but in a fraction of the time. To handle a contraction, a woman must relax completely within a few seconds after it begins, and stay relaxed throughout. She must be able to check her entire body for tension, quickly and easily, over and over. Tell your partner to release these four points:

Face/neck/shoulders

Hands

Bottom (perineum)/thighs

Feet

To practice:

- Tell your partner to "let go" with specific body parts. Telling her to "relax" may make no sense to her in the middle of a contraction, when her whole body is hard at work.

- As you remind your partner of 4-point releasing, relax your own body. Feel in yourself the looseness you are helping her to work for. It will show in your face and body and in your voice, and will help her to follow you. Keep your voice calm and soothing, even when you are being firm.

Mothers-to-be are often told to wait to start labor breathings until they need them, or until they are uncomfortable with walking and talking during a contraction. During early labor, until this point is reached, tension builds up. Accumulated tension causes a woman to start with one strike against her. To avoid this, you should think of relaxation as a dependable friend to call on from the start. The mild Braxton-Hicks contractions felt during late pregnancy offer your partner a perfect chance to practice. Your partner—and you, too—will use the 4-point releasing most easily if you practice it regularly and frequently, and make it part of your daily lives, using it for everyday upsets as well.

□ □ □

"Sue and I did the breathings with each contraction and BOTH tried to relax. From Monday morning until the baby was born Tuesday afternoon I was awake, and we both needed to relax when time permitted."

□ □ □

With special breathings (see the following pages), if it is hard to coordinate releasing with breathing, tell your partner to let go of an area every time she exhales:

"In...out (release face/neck/shoulders)"
"In...out (release hands)"
"In...out (release bottom and thighs)"
"In...out (release feet)"

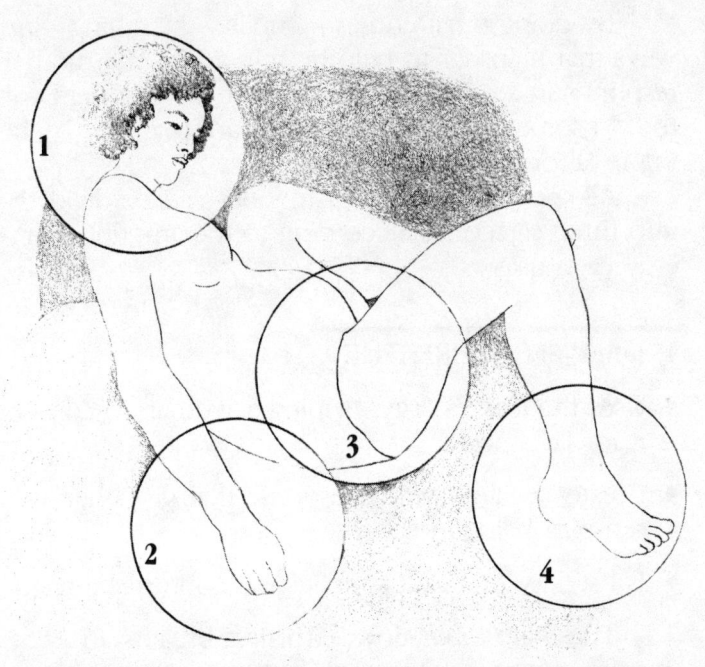

4-point releasing: In a comfortable position, relax these 4 points. They are shortcuts to total relaxation. The rest of your body will follow along. Breathe naturally. Concentrate on letting go of tension

BREATHING

When a mother uses special breathings in labor, she helps both herself and her baby.

Instead of holding her breath or breathing fast and unevenly, as people do when they are nervous or in pain, a mother makes it a point to breathe slowly and evenly. This way she gives herself and her baby plenty of oxygen. Also, she avoids becoming hyperventilated (for details on hyperventilation, see page 235), the result of irregular, deep, fast breathing.

By doing what comes naturally—breathing—in ways that help her to help herself, a laboring mother responds in a constructive way to her inner demands to "do something," demands that are triggered by being in labor.

All special breathing techniques can be divided into three categories, according to the amount of energy each uses.

1. DEEP SLOW BREATHING

- Uses the least energy, helping a woman to conserve it for later needs.

- Creates a calm, steady response that gives her a sense of being in control.

- Is used as long as it supplies the control she needs.

These are long, slow, effortless breaths, in through the nose, out through the mouth.

To practice:

- When she breathes in through her nose, your partner should use as little effort as possible. Suggest that she think of her breath floating lightly into her body, filling up her lungs almost under its own power.

- Next, she should blow out the air slowly and softly, as though whistling silently through gently pursed lips.

Your partner's neck and shoulders may tighten up, especially as she inhales. Watch them. Touch them. Remind her to keep them loose all the time. Remember the other relaxing points as well.

SUGGESTIONS FOR SLOW BREATHING

- **If her nose is stuffy, all breathing can be done through the mouth.** Tell her to place her tongue just behind her teeth, on the the roof of her mouth, and part her lips only a little, just enough to let the air in and out easily. Use Chapstick or Vaseline for dry lips.

- **Keep the breaths even.** If breathing in takes a little longer than breathing out does, she slowly fills up with un-exhaled air until she feels tight and tense. If exhalations are longer, she slowly empties of air until she needs to take a huge deep breath. Use your hand or finger to conduct her through breathing, just as a conductor would conduct an orchestra. Raise your hand as she inhales, lower it as she exhales. Or nod your head, up as she inhales, down as she exhales. Adjust your pace to hers.

- **Think of this breathing as though it were going around in a continuously moving circle:** *in*, up and over the top; *out*, down and around the bottom; *in*, back up; and so on. Keep it moving slowly and easily.

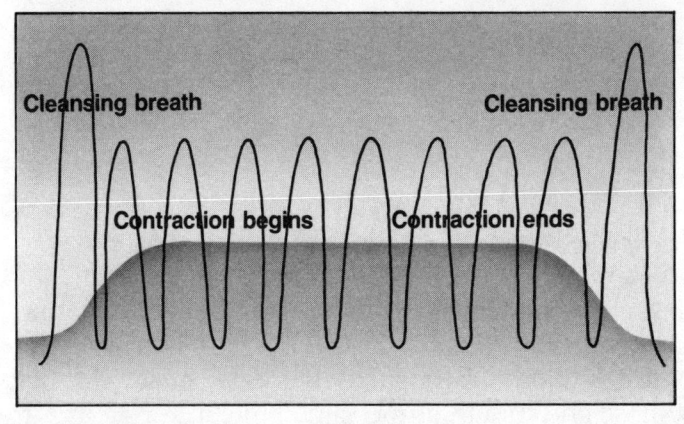

Slow Breathing

- **Remember that this breathing is deep, so it must be slow.** A safe rate is 9 or fewer breaths per minute, not counting the cleansing breaths. To slow down to this rate, concentrate on *easy, gentle* breaths, with the body very loose. Avoid forcing longer breaths. And avoid holding the breath before inhaling and exhaling—two ways people may try to slow down. These *do slow down breathing, but they also create tension.*

> **All breathings are easiest when the body is loose.** Remember 4-point releasing. Face, shoulders, and hands often need special attention.

2. QUICK SHALLOW BREATHING

- Uses more energy than long, slow breathing. But shallow breathing also conserves energy because it, too, uses energy carefully and efficiently.

- Supplies a more active response to balance stronger, more active contractions. If kept even and calm, it continues to give a sense of being well in control.

- Is used whenever a woman needs the control it supplies.

These breaths are *short* and *shallow*, done *easily* and *lightly* at the back of the throat or high in the chest. They are done through the mouth, usually, but may be done through the nose if it feels better and control is good. Or they may be done equally through the nose and mouth at the same time. The pace is 5 to

10 breaths over a 5-second period, rather like a dog panting in *slow motion*. Sometimes this breathing is called panting, or mouth-centered breathing. When it speeds up and slows down to match the contraction as it strengthens and weakens, it may be called accelerated/decelerated breathing.

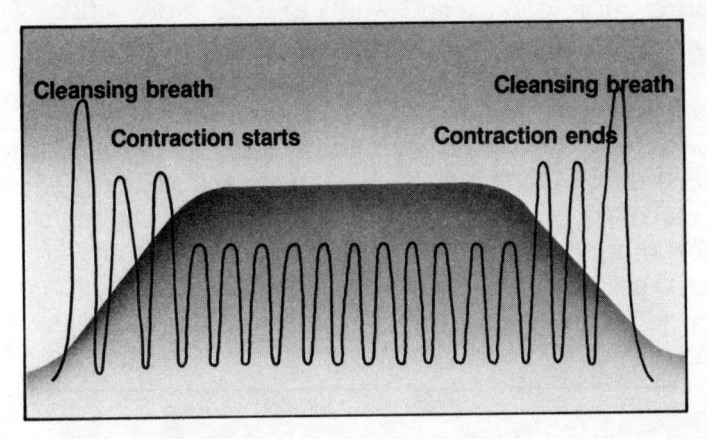

Shallow Breathing

To practice:

- Remind your partner to do the quick, shallow breaths as though whispering the letter "e" very quietly, over and over.

- Inhalation is effortless. Exhalation (when the "e" is whispered) is short and almost bitten off, like a staccato sound in music.

- Watch all 4 releasing points, especially face, neck, and shoulders. These tend to hold tension more than the other 3 areas.

COMBINATION BREATHING

As contractions become stronger your partner may feel that slow breathing is not helping any more, or is helping only for part of the contraction, say the beginning and the end. In the middle or at the peak she needs more control and wants to use a more active breathing. Slow and shallow breathings can be used in combination to match a contraction as it strengthens and weakens. For example, at the start of a contraction the slow breathing could be used as long as it feels right. As the contraction, growing stronger, reaches its peak, a switch to shallow breathing might feel more appropriate. As the contraction lets up, so can the breathing. A return to slow breathing saves energy. For contractions that are strong from the beginning, start with shallow breathing.

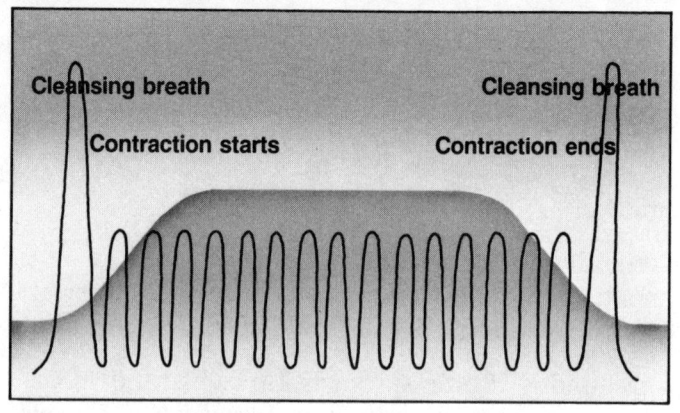

Combination Breathing

□ □ □

"I knew when to use the next breathing exercise, when I couldn't concentrate well enough with the one I was using. Then I would go on to the next. I even went back again a couple of times."

To practice:
Include "changing gears" in the practice of both slow and shallow breathings.

3. EMERGENCY BREATHING

Emergency breathing is quick, shallow breathing in a special pattern.

- Uses more energy than the other two breathings, but still uses it carefully.

- Supplies the most active response—along with the greater concentration needed to follow the special pattern that balances very strong, demanding contractions.

To practice:
Remind your partner to practice this breathing by combining short, shallow panting breaths with short, shallow puffs or blows in a pattern. The panting breaths are done as though whispering the letter "e" over and over, and the puffs are like blowing out a match. The pattern is often 3 pants and 1 puff, or 1 pant and 1 puff. The rhythm is very helpful for dealing with stress.

"e - e - e puff! e - e - e puff!" (3 and 1 breathing)
or
"e - puff! e - puff! e - puff!" (1 and 1 breathing)

The combination may, of course, be any one that helps the most.

In labor, mothers find themselves naturally breathing faster as a contraction grows stronger, and slower as the contraction weakens. This happens even when they have never practiced breathing this way. If you

Emergency Breathings

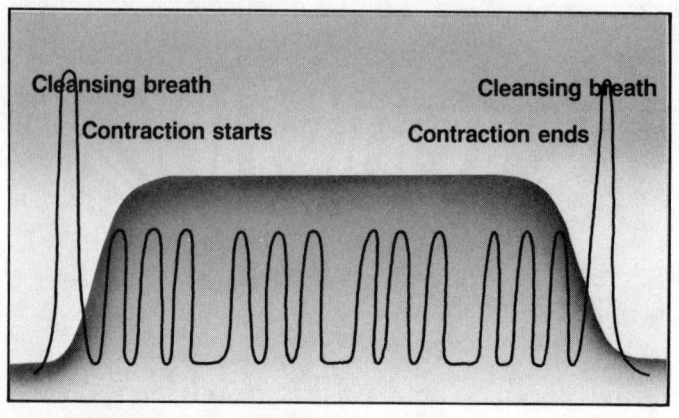

3 & 1 Breathing

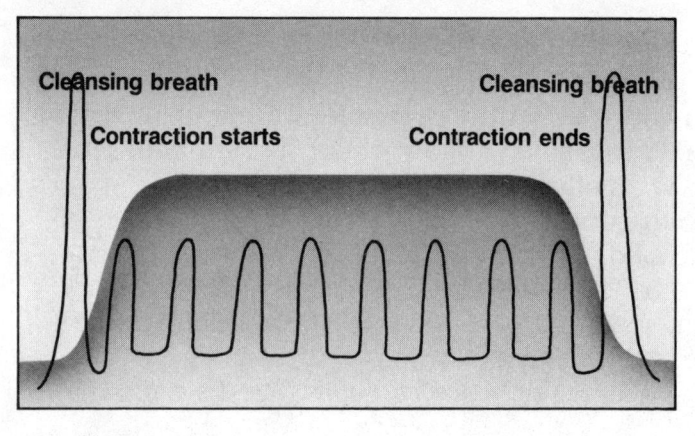

1 & 1 Breathing

practice at your top speed, the pace in labor may become frantic and out of rhythm. This can lead to hyperventilation and loss of control. A slower pace in practice will lead to a slower, easier pace in labor.

- In practice, a workable pace is about 5 to 10 breaths over a 5-second period. Concentrate on the pattern and rhythm of breathing and on 4-point releasing.

- A trick that almost always works to make shallow breathings feel right is to sing them, or hum them on every exhalation, as though singing "e - e - e - e..." over and over. Make sure your partner inhales as usual between each "e".

This advanced breathing is usually called *transition breathing* because it suits the long, strong contractions—typical of transition—that call for extra control. Actually, it helps for any difficult time when extra control is needed. Instead of saving it for transition only, you could think of it as emergency breathing reserved for all rough spots.

Occasionally, puffs are used alone. Uninterrupted puffs or blowing out repeatedly are more likely to cause hyperventilation than are other kinds of breathing. It is easy to make puffs deeper than they should be when they are done over and over without a break. Be careful to remind your partner to keep puffs shallow, with equal amounts of air breathed in and out.

SUGGESTIONS FOR SHALLOW BREATHINGS

Remember:

- **Keep the breaths shallow, even, light, easy.**

- **They should be done as effortlessly as possible**, especially in practice, because breathing will naturally become more pronounced and forceful in labor.

To avoid a **dry mouth**:

- Breathe very quietly. Make inhalations silent and effortless.

- Breathe from the back of the throat, rather than from the front of the mouth.

- Place the tongue behind the front top teeth or on the roof of the mouth.

- Part the lips only a little, just enough to allow air to pass through.

- With the lips parted, breathe through mouth *and* nose, as though humming without sound (try it first with sound, then without).

To break **ragged rhythm**:

- Carefully follow 4-point releasing.

- Slow down.

- Make sure that every exhalation is followed by an inhalation. Breathe in a 4/4 rhythm:
  >OUT-in / OUT-in / OUT-in / OUT-in
  >1-and / 2-and / 3-and / 4-and

  The exhalation gets the downbeat. Accent it.

- Keep your attention on the breathing. Concentrate carefully.

- Interrupt ragged rhythm by taking a quick, shallow breath in through the nose, and releasing it through the mouth, like a sniff followed by a puff—and then continue with the breathing of her choice.

To fight **fatigue**:

- Carefully follow 4-point releasing, especially face/neck/shoulders.

- Keep all breathings easy, light, quiet, even.
- Follow a moderate pace.

To help if your partner feels she is **not getting enough air**:

- Carefully follow 4-point releasing.
- Allow the air that is needed to come in. Make breaths big enough to take in the needed air, keeping them light and even.

WHEN TO CHANGE BREATHINGS

To save energy during labor, it makes sense to use the slow breathing first, for as long as it feels right, and then to go on to the second, and later the third, only when an earlier kind of breathing is no longer helpful. Classes and books often suggest changing from one breathing to another when the cervix reaches a certain dilation. In labor, many women find this impractical, because they do not know at all times how much they are dilated, especially if they are still at home. Many find it easier to tune in to how they feel, using a different breathing when it seems to work better.

To change breathings when a woman feels the need to change may save her more energy than if she struggles to stick with an earlier breathing that isn't working well, merely because it seems too early to switch to another.

□ □ □

"There was little conscious choosing of one breathing technique over another. It just seemed to be a natural progression from one to another as it became necessary."

"I didn't know which to use, so I kept trying all of them until I got one that worked for me."

Sometimes a mother chooses advanced breathing because she is nervous or fearful. Even though contractions themselves are relatively mild, they may seem strong to her. Worried about coping and afraid of pain, she may be trying to shut out what she is feeling by tensing up and breathing rapidly. This struggle makes it hard for her to know what is really going on inside her, and to choose the best way to manage.

- If you think an advanced breathing is being used too soon, suggest an earlier one. Make sure to emphasize 4-point releasing.

In the hospital a nurse may advise you to use an earlier breathing. It is always a sound idea to try out the suggestion. With your encouragement, your partner may find herself comfortable with the suggested breathing.

- First, try it out together between contractions. When the next contraction starts, breathe with her through the whole contraction. For calmness and control, remind her of 4-point releasing as you go.

- After working together for several contractions you both will have a chance to judge which breathing works best.

□ □ □

"Not knowing what the duration of labor was to be, or what the intensity of pain would be, we got to 1 and 1 breathing by midnight. The nurse on duty diplomatically suggested that we return to the chest breathings to conserve her energy."

"I was using shallow breathing all through. One nurse worried, but I knew better."

At this point, if your partner insists that the advanced breathing is the only one that helps, give her the benefit of the doubt and work with her. A mother may feel her labor advancing before anyone else suspects that this is happening. Particularly with mothers who have had babies before, or those whose dilation has reached 5 to 7 centimeters (2½ to 3½ fingers) the cervix can open suddenly and even dilate completely within a few minutes.

□ □ □

"I once tried to correct her method of breathing and was told in no uncertain terms that my advice wasn't needed but that my back-pushing was."

□ □ □

A mother can waste energy if she struggles to use a breathing that does not fit her needs. If a breathing technique is helping her, she will feel more in control, which gives her more confidence. She will be better able to breathe in an energy-saving way—lightly and in rhythm. There is no rule. The right breathing is the one that feels right.

□ □ □

"From our experience, I would say that the main point is for the papa to talk relaxation into the mother, with affectionate hand-holding."

□ □ □

Even in early labor, it is possible to go to advanced breathing for a short time. Temporary situations that are especially hard to manage may need extra control—for instance, a sudden powerful contraction, a rough ride to the hospital, an uncomfortable vaginal exam. (4-point releasing will also help.)

After your partner has used advanced breathing for a temporary trouble spot, remind her to go back to a breathing that matches her progress in labor. Remember that advanced breathing is designed to match active or transitional labor contractions, when progress usually is rapid. If this strenuous breathing is used continuously in early labor, your partner may think she is further along than she actually is. This drains her mental energy. At the same time she is using extra physical energy when it is not yet necessary.

Almost every contraction eases up toward the end. Long slow breathing in the last 15 seconds of a contraction helps to bring the mother down from her intense hard work level. It also helps her to let go of the contraction more fully after the final cleansing breath. You usually can sense when this let-up begins because your partner's efforts become less intense. During the last 15 seconds or so you can say "I think your contraction is letting up. If it feels right to you, change to slow breathing for the end."

□ □ □

"My husband kept telling me how far into each contraction I was, which was a great help. The only thing I could recall anyone saying was '15 seconds, 30, 45, 60—this contraction is over.'"

□ □ □

TIMES WHEN EMERGENCY BREATHING MIGHT BE USED

- During especially powerful contractions.
- During a very uncomfortable vaginal exam.

- When resisting the urge to push if it comes before the cervix is fully dilated, or when the baby is being born.

- When the perineum burns as it stretches during the baby's birth.

- During a manual exam of the inside of the uterus, or when pressure is put on the top of the uterus—both done directly after birth.

PUSHING

During the second stage of labor, mother and uterus actively assist each other to move the baby through her open cervix, down her vagina, and out of her body. When the uterus contracts, the mother pushes.

The urge to push may be felt at various times. It may surprise your partner during transition. It may come suddenly after dilation. Or it may not be felt until several second-stage contractions have passed. Occasionally, a woman never feels it at all. It can come on strongly all at once, or it may start with a little catch in the throat and build up contraction by contraction.

During a contraction it may be present as a steady force to which your partner may respond by pushing steadily throughout the contraction, stopping a few times only to take in a fresh breath of air. Or the urge may come and recede as waves do, to which your partner may respond with a combination of shallow breathing and pushing.

Often the urge is overwhelmingly powerful. Sometimes it is mild and controllable.

Pushing is enormously hard work. Besides concentration, to use her energy to best advantage the mother needs:

1. Good coordination
2. A clear sense of working with her body during contractions
3. Complete rest during breaks

Coordination means combining effort (pushing) with releasing (opening up to let the baby out) both at the same time.

Many mothers find it difficult to open up as they push. They tend to tighten muscles around their vaginas because of pain (from the pressure of the baby), embarrassment or modesty (because their legs are wide open), and anxiety (because it feels as if an enormous bowel movement is about to come out). The power of the pushing urge itself, welling up inside beyond control, is also overwhelming.

If a woman tightens her vagina as she pushes, she works against herself. Pain increases, she hurts more, and the baby's birth takes longer.

To practice:
Once or twice a day, when your partner empties her bladder, she can practice a gentle bearing down. As she sits on the toilet, with her knees wide apart and her hands around her thighs, she can take a deep breath and push gently to make her urine come out as fast as she can. She should feel her abdominal muscles tighten, and the muscles around her vagina bulge outward. She does not need to push hard. In fact, if she strains hard as she pushes, she is likely to think about how hard she is pushing instead of whether she is pushing correctly. If she relaxes her face, and allows her mouth to remain open slightly, she will find it easier to open her bottom. Her legs must be loose also.

Emptying her bladder beforehand, she should

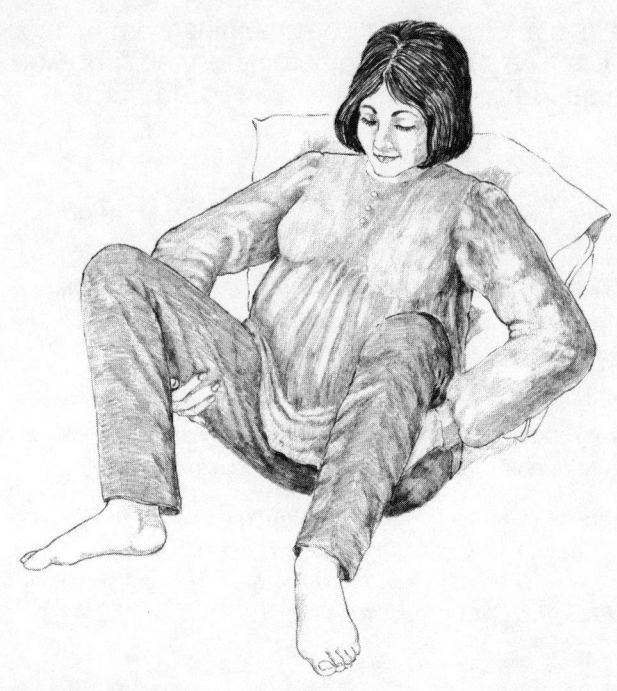

Practicing Pushing

open in the same way when she does her complete pushing practice.

When you practice together, you can place your hand against her perineum, or way down on her lower abomen just above the pubic bone, and ask her to push as though she were trying to push your hand away.

Plenty of practice before labor starts, and supportive coaching when she pushes during labor, help a mother to help her baby out instead of holding back.

If she gets used to these feelings in practice, she can transfer them to pushing with contractions in labor. It is a lot easier to do something from memory than it is to try to learn something on the spot. You can remind her: "Push just as you did in practice."

□ □ □

"Maria's face looked like she had just plugged her finger into an electric socket."

"I have never felt such an urge in my whole life. It's quite a fantastic feeling when they let you push, and the pain is negligible."

"Pushing seemed really intense, almost orgasmic. I believe because Jennifer initiated the push, then let the sensation take over, she had a very productive and rewarding pushing."

"I found pushing to be the most difficult and painful part of labor. I would start pushing as soon as I felt the urge, but I lost the urge somewhere in the middle of the contraction and found it difficult to return to my breathing."

□ □ □

Effective pushing requires:

1. Knowing how to push
2. Knowing how to open up—at the same time
3. A workable position

PUSHING TECHNIQUE AS IT IS COMMONLY TAUGHT

1. One or two cleansing breaths (see page 23) before and after a pushing contraction supply extra oxygen and help the mother to ease into and out of her work.

2. After the beginning cleansing breaths, your partner will take in another breath, hold it, bring her head forward, and push, for as long as she can.

3. At the end of this push, with her head back, she quickly blows out and inhales again. She brings her head forward again, and pushes some more.

4. These steps are repeated several times as needed until the contraction is over. Then she takes the cleansing breaths that signal her rest time.

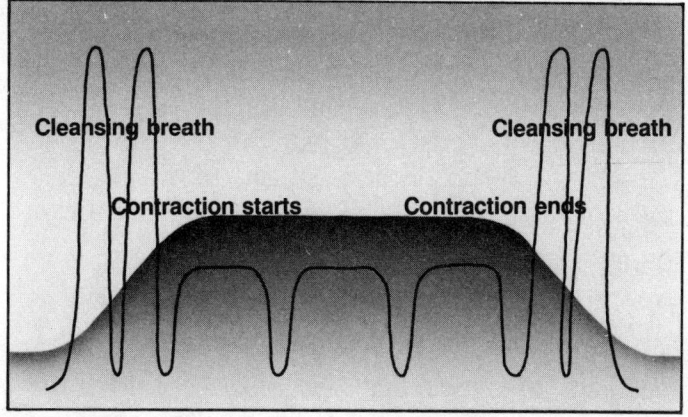

Pushing Breathing

◻ ◻ ◻

"Because we had practiced so little, Alison had no idea how to push. She also did not know how to get a fresh gulp of air between pushes. And I wasn't sure how to help her. Luckily the nurse breathed with her a few times."

◻ ◻ ◻

VARIATIONS ON PUSHING TECHNIQUE

These are beginning to be taught because they are closer to the way many women experience labor.

> **Note:** Because the midwife or doctor will have the final word about the way your partner's delivery is handled, be sure you both exchange ideas with her or him during the pregnancy. Understanding one another is important. Knowing that your midwife or doctor supports your goals helps if a last-minute change in plans is necessary. A big baby, for example, or one who is in trouble and needs to be born as soon as possible may call for an all-out pushing effort instead of the gentler approach described here.

- **During a push**, your partner lets a little air slowly slip out through her lips, or sighs it out through her throat. At the end of the push, she blows out the remaining air, then inhales again for the next push.

- **During a contraction, between pushes**, she inhales smoothly at a leisurely pace, as fast or as slowly as she feels is comfortable.

- **One push, or several, may be sprinkled through a contraction**, depending on what the mother is feeling. During a contraction, a woman pushes only when she feels the urge. She continues to push as long as pushing feels productive. Otherwise she uses her choice of the shallow breathings.

- Although a woman can push with her arms relaxed, **if more force is needed it helps to grasp something.** Side rails, hand grips, stirrup bars, or arms of attendants are better to pull on than her own legs. Legs tend to tighten up and, in turn, so does the perineum. This also may happen if she pushes her feet against something like the foot of the bed or footrests on stirrups.

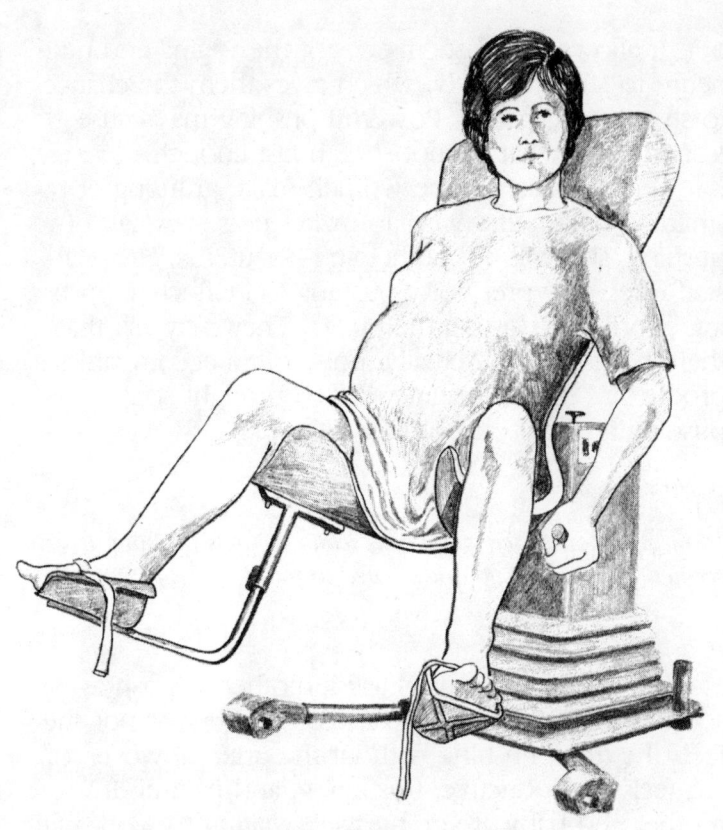

It helps to grasp something when you push

- If a woman does **no-push breathing when she feels her perineum burning**, the uterus pushing alone permits the vagina and perineum to stretch slowly.

  Gentle pushing keeps oxygen at a higher level for both mother and baby. With it, a woman saves energy and so is less tired. It lessens strain on her face and neck. Blowing out a little stream of air while pushing makes it easier for her to use her abdominal muscles correctly, pulling them in, instead of pushing them out. It allows the elastic tissues of the vagina and perineum to stretch slowly, which gives them the chance to stretch to capacity. Powerful pushing may cause tears in tissue that cannot stretch fast enough.

As they push, some women make grunting or straining noises. If a woman makes noise *instead* of pushing, she will not be helping her uterus. Hospital staff often interpret noisy pushing as ineffective pushing effort, or "wasting the push." They may ask that there be no noise. Actually, noise often accompanies a productive effort. Imagine how you might sound pushing a heavy car out of a ditch.

□ □ □

"Sandra let out a few good yells while she was pushing. It seemed to help and no one seemed to mind."

□ □ □

Medical attendants usually ask a mother to push as soon as the cervix is fully dilated, whether or not she feels the urge. Pushing without the urge, however, often feels unproductive, frustrating, and painful. If mother and baby are doing well, waiting to work with the pushing urge may feel most comfortable and natural. Slow or shallow breathing can be used with contractions until pushing begins, or between pushes if the urge comes and goes in surges.

- Your approach to pushing may be different from what the hospital staff tells you to do. It makes a difference if you have discussed your ideas beforehand with your doctor and received his or her agreement to try them. Explain this to the staff. Ask them to help you try your ideas for the next few contractions at least, to see how they work. On the other hand, your partner and you may feel more comfortable following their instructions.

If pushes are too short to move the baby along, and the staff is asking for longer pushes, you can start counting aloud when your partner starts each push.

- Count **slowly** to 6, to time a 10-second push for her. She may then push on her own, or you may need to continue counting for each push. Of course she can push beyond your count if it feels right to her.

HOW TO KEEP FROM PUSHING

Most times, the urge to push starts shortly before or right after the cervix is open wide enough (10 centimeters or 5 fingers) to allow the baby to come through easily. The urge can be overwhelmingly powerful. There are times when your partner will be told not to push, to allow the uterus to work alone for slower and gentler progress. For example, this might happen during transition, or while waiting for the doctor, or on the way to the delivery room, or during the baby's birth.

▫ ▫ ▫

"At the risk of sounding big-headed let me say had it not been for me counting and breathing with her, she would have given birth 20 minutes before the doctor arrived."

▫ ▫ ▫

Panting or puffing is an effective way for a woman to resist pushing when her urge is powerful. Instead of using the pushing force, she releases it by blowing or breathing it out. The control it takes to puff instead of push is enormous. When the nurse, midwife, or doctor asks your partner to wait to push, or to stop pushing, the no-push breathing must be an automatic response. She is working too hard to take time out to think what to do. It must be built-in, like putting your foot on the brake of a car when you see a red light. This comes only with a lot of practice.

□ □ □

"I kept telling everyone I couldn't control it, though the blowing did."

□ □ □

No-Push Breathing

To practice:
Because your partner cannot practice with the urge itself, she must learn to respond to the words she is most likely to hear in labor: "Don't push" or "Stop pushing." Every time you say "Don't push" or "Stop pushing" (and she can say it to herself when she practices alone), she should pant-blow (or whatever breathing she prefers for this control). Using these words, interrupt her as she practices breathing and as she

practices pushing. After a while she will respond without having to think it out each time, and it will be easier for her to follow these instructions in labor.

POSITIONS FOR BIRTH

Pushing may take an hour or two, occasionally longer, especially for a first-time mother or for a large or posterior baby. The mother may want to use one position to move her baby down to her vaginal opening and another during the 5 to 15 minutes of giving birth.

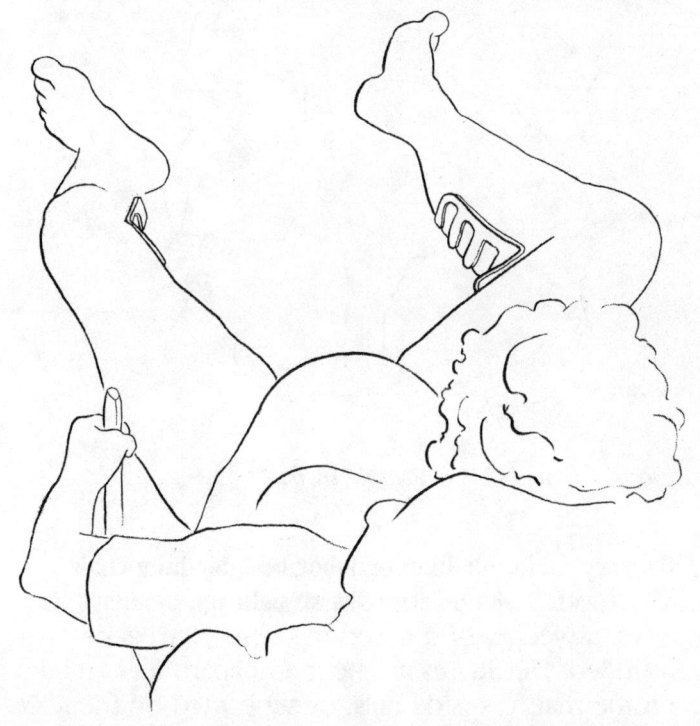

Positions for birth: At an angle on delivery table, with stirrups

These birthing positions are listed in the order most commonly used in hospitals in the United States, preferred by most obstetricians here.

1. **Delivery table, birthing or labor bed, birthing chair.** The mother is **on her back, flat or at an angle** against pillows, wedge, or raised mattress. Her legs rest in stirrups. Her hands hold hand grips or stirrup bars, or rest on the mattress. The birthing chair, in which a mother may lie or sit, is owned by only a few hospitals.

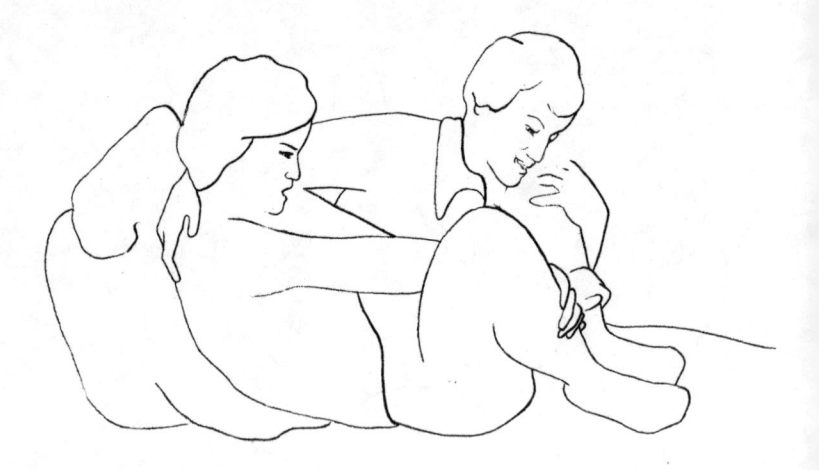

Positions for birth: At an angle in bed

2. **Delivery table, birthing or labor bed, birthing chair.** The mother **sits or semi-sits straight up,** against pillows, a wedge, or a raised mattress. Her back is rounded. Her knees are bent and apart, legs resting on the mattress, side rails, or supported by friends. Her hands hold her legs, hand grips, side rails, or friends, hands, or rest on the mattress.

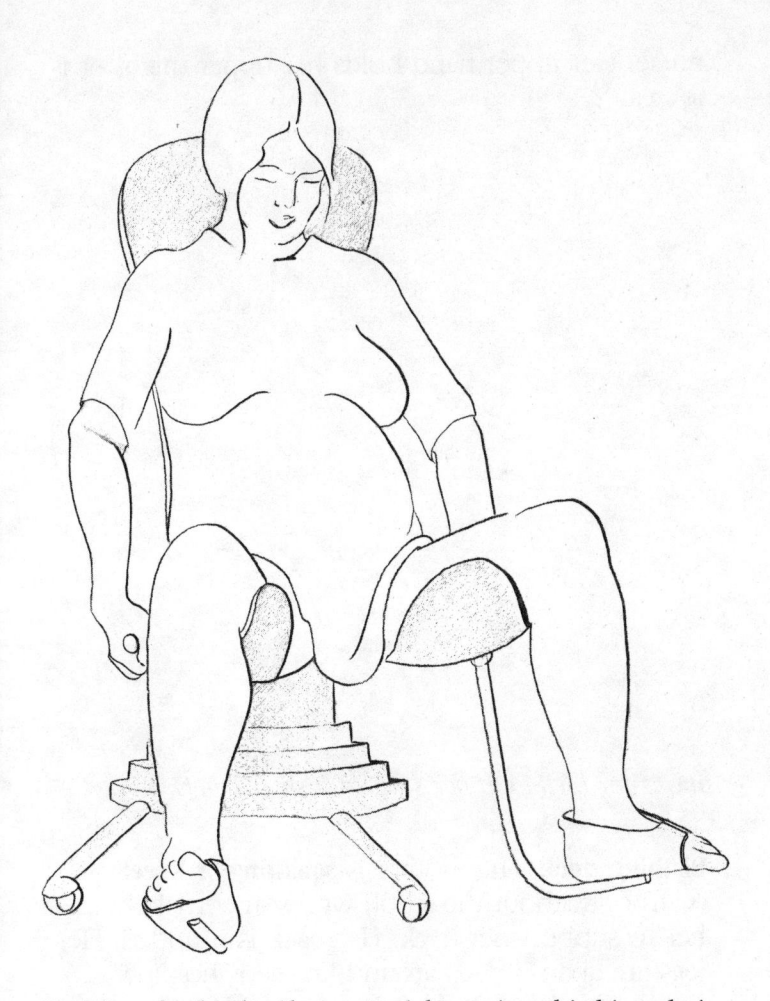

Positions for birth: Almost straight up in a birthing chair

3. **Delivery table, birthing or labor bed.** The mother is **on her side, flat or at a slight angle,** with a pillow under her head. Her back is rounded. Her knees are bent with her upper leg raised and resting on a side rail padded with a pillow or supported by you or a

nurse. Her upper hand holds her upper thigh, or is at rest.

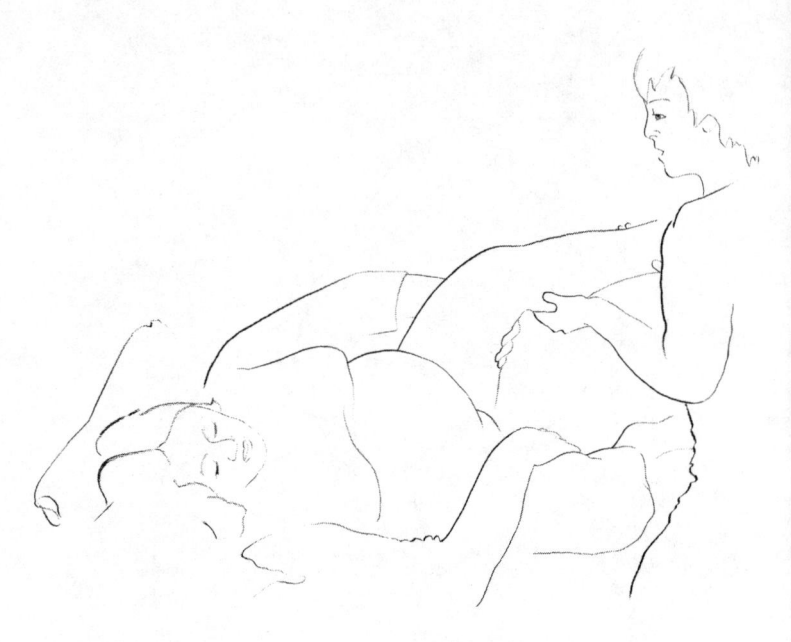

Positions for birth: On her side, at a slight angle, in bed

4. **Birthing stool:** The mother is **squatting or kneeling** (with or without the stool) with someone behind her to support her back. Her back is rounded. Her legs are apart, hands around knees or holding something for support (table, bed, side rail).

5. **Delivery table, birthing or labor bed** (in the lowest position near the floor, with the side rails up for safety), **or floor** (clean and padded with clean sheets). The mother is on her **hands and knees**. Her back is rounded, or her head and arms may rest on a chair, or bed.

POSITIONS FOR BIRTH 57

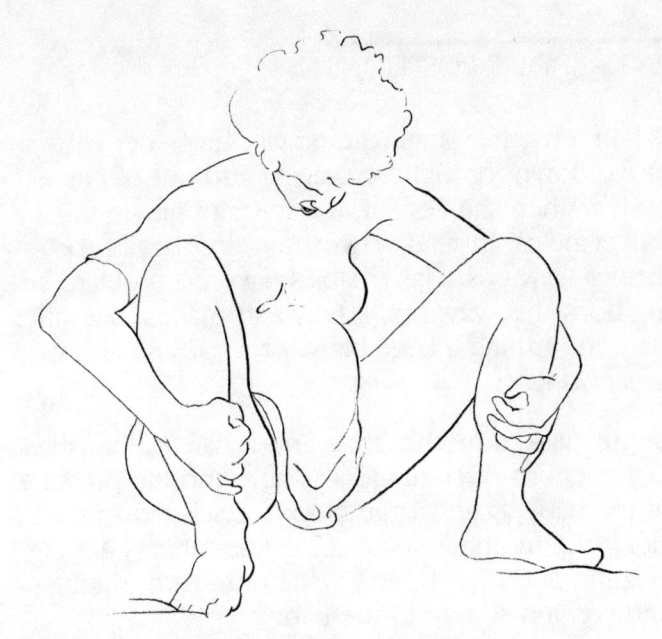

Positions for birth: Squatting

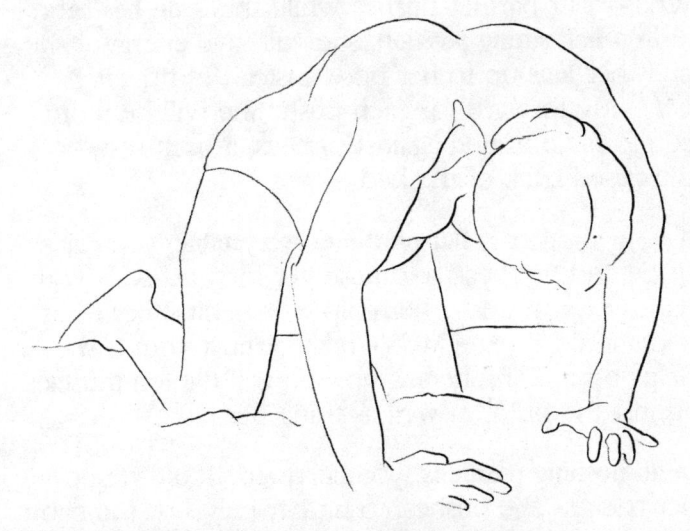

Positions for birth: On her hands and knees

POINTS ABOUT POSITIONS

- When a mother is **upright**, gravity helps her baby to move down through her vagina and out of her body. When she lies flat, the force of gravity no longer helps. Instead, it works against her as she pushes upwards. Many babies have no problem being born this way, but gravity can make a big difference in birthing a large baby, or a baby in an unusual position.

- **On her back**, a mother may find it hard to breathe. Contractions often are less strong, and the pressure of the baby against large blood vessels that run along the mother's spine sometimes affects her circulation and blood pressure (and, in turn, the blood and oxygen supply to the baby).

- When your partner pushes while she is **on her back, or in a half-sitting position**, she will save energy if she pulls her legs up to her body instead of bringing her body forward for each push. She will be more comfortable resting against pillows, a back rest, or the raised back of the bed.

- If your partner is **flat on the delivery table**, you can sit behind her head and raise her forward with your hands or arm under her pillow or behind her head and shoulders. She MUST relax against you. If she helps by holding herself up, she will tighten muscles against the birth, as well as tiring herself.

- **In all pushing positions**, your partner should round her back as she pushes, to tilt her pelvis so the baby can move through it more easily.

To practice:
Practice pushing in several positions. You cannot know in advance which will be most comfortable for your partner or best suited to moving the baby along. A large baby may make better progress if her mother is in an upright pushing position because gravity helps to bring the baby down. A baby in a posterior position, pressing on the mother's back (see Back Labor, page 244), may move forward into a more workable position when the mother pushes on her side or on her hands and knees. A baby being born too rapidly can be slowed for a gentler, more controlled delivery when a mother lies on her side.

THE IMPORTANCE OF PRACTICE

For relaxing, for breathing, and for pushing, you and your partner *must* practice. Her skills *and* your skills need to be second nature. They will become second nature only when they are done over and over. In the midst of hard, demanding work it is difficult to think, and to make and carry through decisions. It isn't enough to understand a technique. Each skill has to become a working response, part of you, a habit that is stronger than logic, theory, or idea. Repeated practice creates that built-in response.

□ □ □

"Without preparation I think I would not have been able to cope as well as I did. Practicing sometimes became very tedious but I made myself plod through them. And having practiced over and over, my body just seemed to know what breathing to use."

"Practicing at home, I felt it was all a waste of time and that

in real labor Vikki would panic. But she didn't, and I didn't, and we did very well."

"It took some work to maintain the systems we had practiced. I thought we had practiced fairly well, but I guess there is no way to practice too much."

□ □ □

SUGGESTIONS FOR PRACTICE

- **Practice at least 3 times a day**, sometimes by yourselves, sometimes together. Keep your sessions short, so you won't get tired or bored. Almost always you can find 10 minutes somewhere in each day.

- **Practice under ideal conditions**—quiet, comfortable, without interference—when you can concentrate most easily so that you can get the most out of your work.

- **After you both have confidence in a certain skill, practice it some of the time with distractions**—noise, other people around you, in different positions, in different places—where it is harder to concentrate. Realistically, conditions and surroundings in labor will present the same challenges. The more at ease both of you are in different situations, the better prepared you will be.

- **If your partner has a problem with a skill, work on it 2 or 3 times** in any one session, and then let it go until you practice next. Harping on a problem creates tension and worry rather than helping it to come out right.

Practice need not be drudgery, something to be

fought because it "should" be done. Keep it interesting, challenging, and fun.

For example: Switch roles. For the mother-to-be, acting as coach can help her to understand how to direct herself through labor. A coach who tries out relaxing, breathing, and pushing, experiences to some degree how these skills feel. Each role is seen from another point of view. When your partner coaches you, she can show you how she likes to be coached. This often gets across the idea more clearly than if she told you.

Practice alone. You both will see your skills differently when you work without one another. Each of you may take your work more seriously. Concentration improves. Certain details are clearer. Effective ways of working—or problems—that were hidden before may show up now. And, very important, your partner will gain confidence that she can work by herself if you should be separated at any time during labor. When you practice your partner's skills, talk to yourself the same way you talk to her when you are coaching her. What gives you the best results when you coach yourself? What problems do you run into? Use the insights to make your coaching more understanding and effective.

Change positions. Stand, sit, kneel, lie down. Your partner can practice on her side, half-sitting, semi-reclining, on hands and knees, squatting, leaning on things—tables, the bed, the wall, against you. Any or all of these positions might be useful in labor.

Practice on the spur of the moment as well as at scheduled times each day. Practice in different situations—in bed, at the movies, while shopping, at work, visiting friends, eating out, in the car. The reality is that labor can take place—and does—under all kinds of circumstances. When labor begins you will feel more confident, knowing that you can use your techniques under various conditions. Remember you also will need the quiet, comfortable practices to give you a chance to concentrate on doing all techniques properly.

When you and your partner work together over several weeks, you become a team, with a greater understanding of how to help each other and how the variations on the techniques may fit your personal needs. You have prepared yourselves to work with labor.

A Quick Guide to Mother's Labor Skills

The 3 basic labor skills are:

- **Relaxing**
- **Breathing**
- **Pushing**

Aids for working with these skills are **Concentration**, **Focus**, and the **Cleansing Breaths**.

Concentration keeps energy and attention centered on working with labor.

Focus, resting eyes on a specific point, prevents visual distractions that interfere with concentration.

Opening the eyes keeps the focus outward. Closing them often causes the focus to turn inward on pain and anxiety, and shuts out helpers like the coach.

The **Cleansing Breaths** isolate each contraction.

With one cleansing breath, the mother greets the contraction at its beginning, declaring her readiness to work.

With another cleansing breath, she lets go of the contraction at its end, turning her attention to other things.

For a cleansing breath, air is inhaled through the nose, blown out through the mouth.

RELAXING

- Saves energy
- Creates calm
- Helps a mother to work with, instead of against, labor

Relaxing is a conscious, disciplined effort acquired with a lot of practice.

Head-to-toe relaxing is a way to learn and practice relaxing.

It is used to get to sleep during pregnancy, and in early labor.

4-point releasing is a short-cut to full relaxation.

It is a labor tool, used on its own to work with contractions and as a foundation for all breathings.

It is used to rest between contractions.

BREATHINGS

- Give mother and baby oxygen
- Are tools to help the mother use her labor energy to work with her body
- Vary in pattern and rhythm to match the changing strength of contractions

> **Deep** breathing must be **slow** breathing.
> **Rapid** breathing must be **shallow** breathing.
> All breathings are even, gentle, rhythmical.

Slow breathing:

- The inhalation "floats" in through the nose.
- The exhalation "whistles" silently out through pursed lips.

Shallow breathings are done through the mouth, from the back of the throat.

- They are shallow, quiet, effortless.
- A 4/4 rhythm can be used to keep the pace even.

Combination breathings are used during some contractions. Slow breathing switches to shallow breathing and back to slow breathing, to match the contraction's changing strength while saving energy.

- Breathing adapts to match a mother's needs.

No-push breathing, or shallow breathing is used to keep from responding to the pushing urge when the midwife or doctor requests that your partner wait to push or stop pushing.

PUSHING

Pushing feels best and is most effective when a mother works with her uterus, bearing down when she feels the urge, allowing herself to open up as she pushes outward through her body and her vagina.

Points to remember about the position for pushing:

- Head forward
- Mouth relaxed
- Shoulders rounded
- Arms rounded
- Abdominal muscles in use (contracted)
- Bottom (perineum) loose and open

Pushing coordination with a contraction (variations included):

- One or 2 cleansing breaths at the start of a contraction, as the mother waits to push with the peak of her pushing urge.
- One or more cleansing breaths at the end of a contraction to give the mother oxygen and to help her to relax.
- Pushing during the contraction may be constant, broken only by air exchanges. Or it may be intermittent as the urge ebbs and flows, interspersed with shallow breathing.
- Breath may be held, or released slowly, perhaps with sound, during the pushes.

PRACTICE OF ALL SKILLS IS ABSOLUTELY ESSENTIAL.

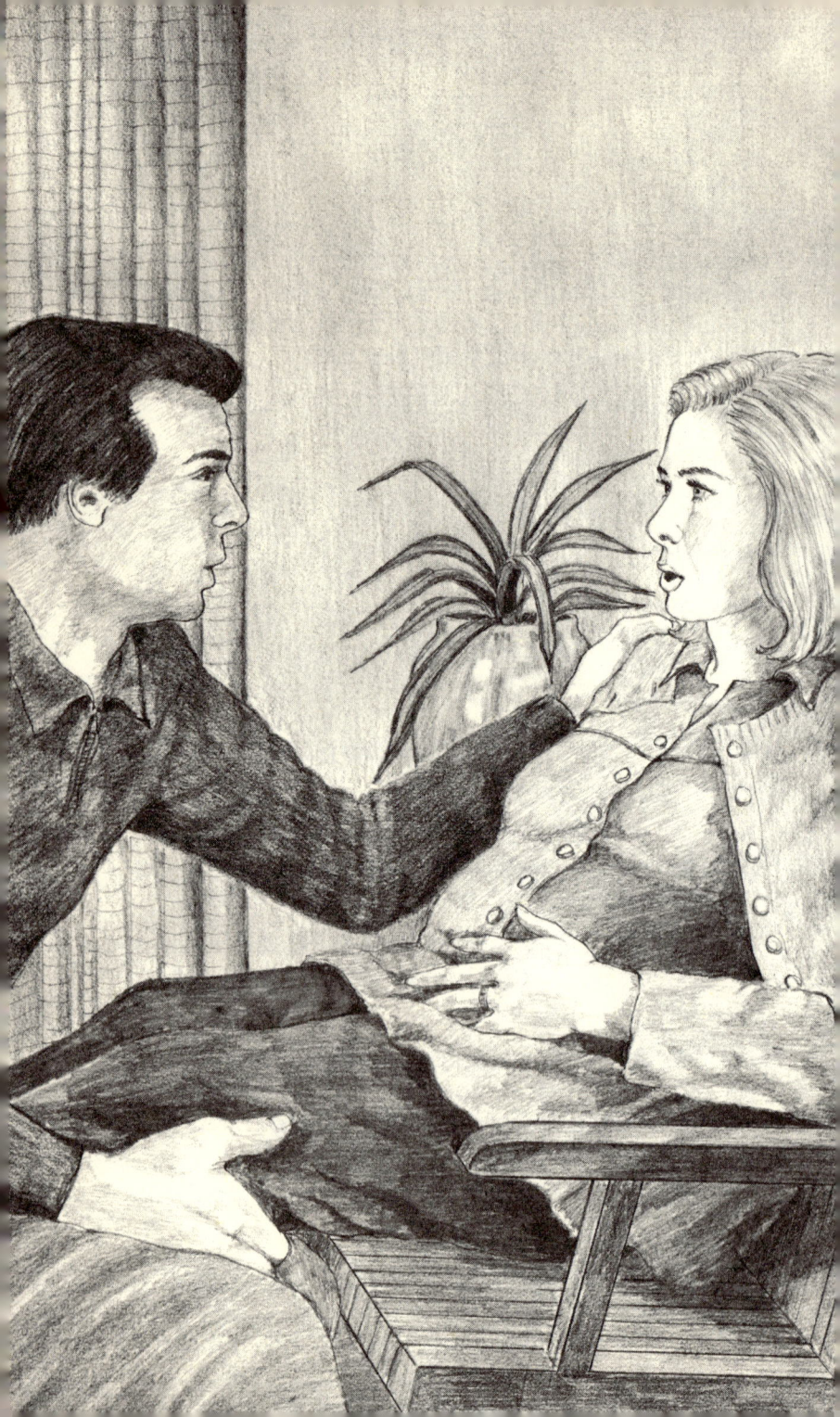

4. Waiting for Labor to Start

Your partner's due date isn't far away. You have finished your childbirth classes. What do you do now?

Waiting is the main activity. There is a lot of waiting when a baby is about to arrive—waiting for labor to begin; next, waiting to know if it *is* labor; and then waiting during labor for its end and the baby's birth.

KEEPING SANE AND PREPARED

Time will pass. The baby *will* be born. The pregnancy *won't* last forever. For the moment, give yourself over to the waiting. Focus on the present. The days seem to move more slowly if you keep a close eye on the calendar. Keep busy to help time pass easily. Continue to practice. It is tempting to slack off, but staying well rehearsed is so important during this home stretch. Also make sure that both you and your partner stay well rested and well nourished.

Keep busy:

- **Plan small projects.** Tour your hospital, if you haven't already (or do it again). Most hospitals have special tour times for which you can sign up. If your tour is cancelled because someone is in labor, or for any other reason, ask if you may come during a non-tour time. Your due date may arrive before a scheduled tour time is open. Evenings are usually less busy for the staff than days. Bring a list of questions when you take the tour. A very complete list is on page 287.

- **Map out 2 or 3 routes to the hospital**, in case one is blocked when you go. Find out where to enter the hospital. Is there a different entrance at night? Where can you park your car?

- **Pack bags** at least 2 weeks before the date your baby is due, or make lists so that you can pack easily at the last minute. Packing the bag while referring to the list might be one of the ways you, as coach, can help during early labor. See the Labor Kit on page 295 for a list of useful items to take, to keep by you during labor.

Keep practicing:

- **Take a refresher lesson** if 2 or 3 weeks have passed since class ended and you are still waiting. An extra class helps to motivate you to practice and to reassure you that you are not alone as you wait.

- **Practice 3 times a day**, together and separately. Use short sessions (15 minutes or so) with lots of concentration and relaxing as a foundation, rather than long sessions that may become boring and sloppy.

Stay well rested: If your partner finds it impossible to sleep through the night, she can try daytime naps. Her 4-point releasing will help to make full use of rest periods. As much as possible, try to stay loose and easy all the time.

Stay well nourished: Labor is hard physical work, like an athletic event. A long-distance runner wouldn't spend the final days before a big event existing on Cokes and munchies. If big meals are not appealing to your partner, suggest that she eat nourishing little ones scattered throughout the day.

Last-minute thoughts: You and your partner still may be having some last-minute pangs over differences of opinion between you and your midwife, doctor, or hospital—even though you have settled finally upon them. At this late date, focus on the pluses, not the minuses—that is, on what you have, rather than on what you don't have. A positive outlook now will help you to feel relaxed and ready. If your feelings have become very strong, however, it is possible to change your midwife or doctor at this late date. First, talk with the person of your choice to make sure she or he can take you on. Then, tell the person you have been seeing so that your records can be transferred.

To be well prepared, you should be ready for as many possibilities as you can. For example, your midwife or doctor may have a group practice or may work at more than one hospital. Recognize the very real possibility that you could end up with an attendant or a hospital that you don't especially like. Learn the facts about Cesareans, forceps, medications, and anesthesia (read Chapter 12, *What to Expect with Variations in Labor,* beginning on page 235). Although these are things you hope will not be part of your experience, they might be. You will be more able to cope with an unexpected situation if you have faced it squarely ahead of time. Being realistic is part of being prepared.

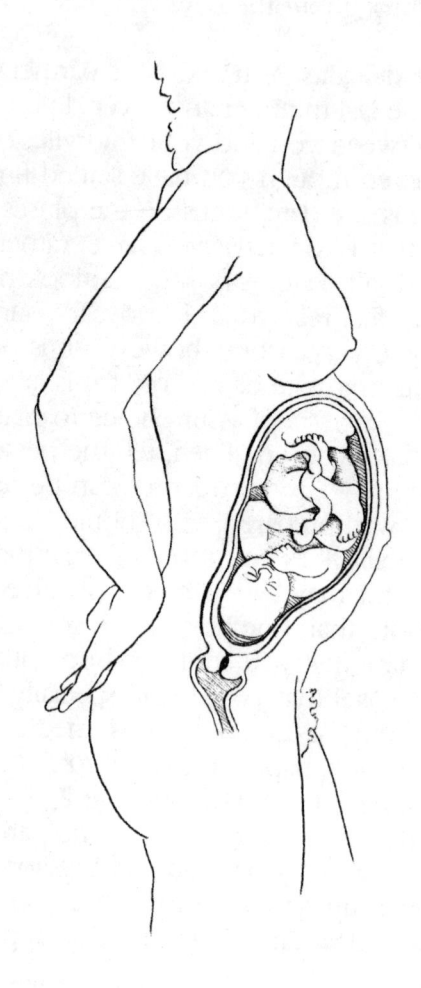

Uterus, with mucus plug

HAS LABOR BEGUN?

Sometimes it is obvious that labor has begun. Sometimes you don't know for sure. You are looking for one of three signs that may appear in any order, close together or spaced widely apart. These signs are:

- The **mucus plug** or **bloody show**
- The **breaking of the bag of water**
- The beginning of **contractions**

THE MUCUS PLUG

The mucus plug, the "cork" inside the cervix, may slip out the day labor begins, or a few days before. It is usually seen as a small mass of clear or whitish mucus. Its passing is easy to overlook. Bloody show (small amounts of pink or red-tinged mucus) does not always mean that labor has begun. Because the cervix bleeds easily in the ninth month, there may be spotting after love-making or a vaginal exam on a routine office visit. Bloody show that signals the beginning of labor may appear once, or on and off. There may be large or small amounts.

□ □ □

"I had no bloody show except for two drops of blood."

"... slight vaginal bleeding, both brown and red throughout the day."

"Instead of blood-tinged mucus it was more like heavy menstrual flow."

THE BAG OF WATER

Perhaps your partner is passing fluid, apparently from her vagina. Is there a break in the water-filled sac surrounding the baby? Or is pressure from the baby causing your partner's bladder to leak urine? Or are the mucus glands of the cervix, superactive during pregnancy, especially productive today?

It is easier to tell if the water bag has broken when the fluid appears as a gush rather than a small leak. Urine and mucus are not apt to gush. Periodic leaking, however, is harder to identify. Once the bag has broken, water will continue to leak out every few minutes. Occasionally the opening in the bag seals itself and then the leaking stops.

"Water" (*amniotic fluid*) from the bag normally is clear or milky with a faint sweet smell. It is slightly sticky. Sometimes bits of vernix (nature's yellow-white skin cream for the baby) are floating in it.

Urine is yellow, and has a familiar odor. Usually, it does not leak every few minutes.

Mucus from a cervix that is not dilating in labor is clear or whitish, and may be thick or thin.

A sure test is to wet a strip of Nitrazine paper in the fluid around the vagina. (Nitrazine paper is sold in most drugstores. Your midwife or doctor, or the hospital labor room, always has some in stock.) Amniotic fluid will change the color of this yellow paper to blue. With urine or vaginal secretions the color will not change.

□ □ □

"I heard a strange noise—kind of like a cork popping from a bottle."

"I felt a trickle. Half an hour later there was another, bigger trickle and the liquid met the test for amniotic fluid. That night, the water really did break—conveniently on the kitchen floor."

"... a slight seepage. We were told to call the doctor when her water broke, but we expected more."

□ □ □

> **Note: If the fluid has an olive-green tinge, be sure to tell your midwife or doctor.** This is probably meconium, the bowel movement of a newborn, normally not passed by the baby until after birth. Meconium is passed in the uterus if the baby is under stress. Often the stress is temporary and a cause for observation rather than worry. The midwife or doctor will ask you both to come to the hospital so that a close check can be kept on the baby until birth, to tell whether the problem is repeated, and, if it is, to decide what to do. The solution could be the induction of labor (see page 250), or a Cesarean (see page 252).

If your partner and you know, or even suspect, that the bag of water has broken, call your midwife or doctor. The bag is a barrier against bacteria. When the barrier no longer exists, bacteria may enter the uterus and cause infection. Your partner may be asked to come to the hospital where she can be closely watched while waiting for contractions to start, as they usually do within a few hours. If her uterus is ready

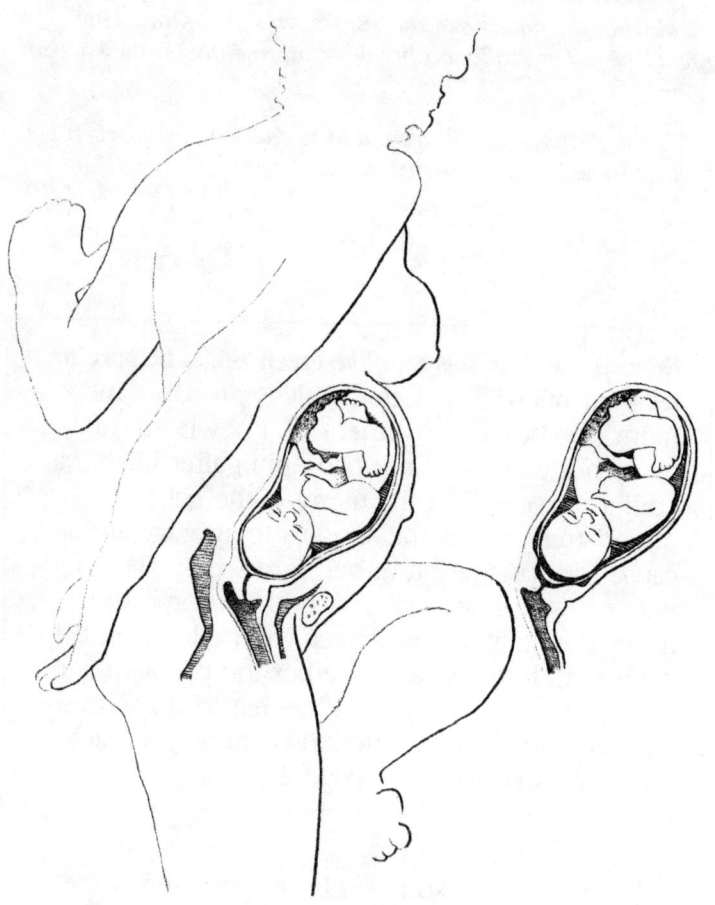

Changes in the cervix, the opening in the uterus, during labor. Left to right, the first three drawings show it effacing, or flattening. The second three drawings show the cervix

for labor—that is, if the cervix is somewhat flattened and open, and the baby has dropped well into the pelvis—contractions may be started artificially (induced). (Please read about induced labor on page 250).

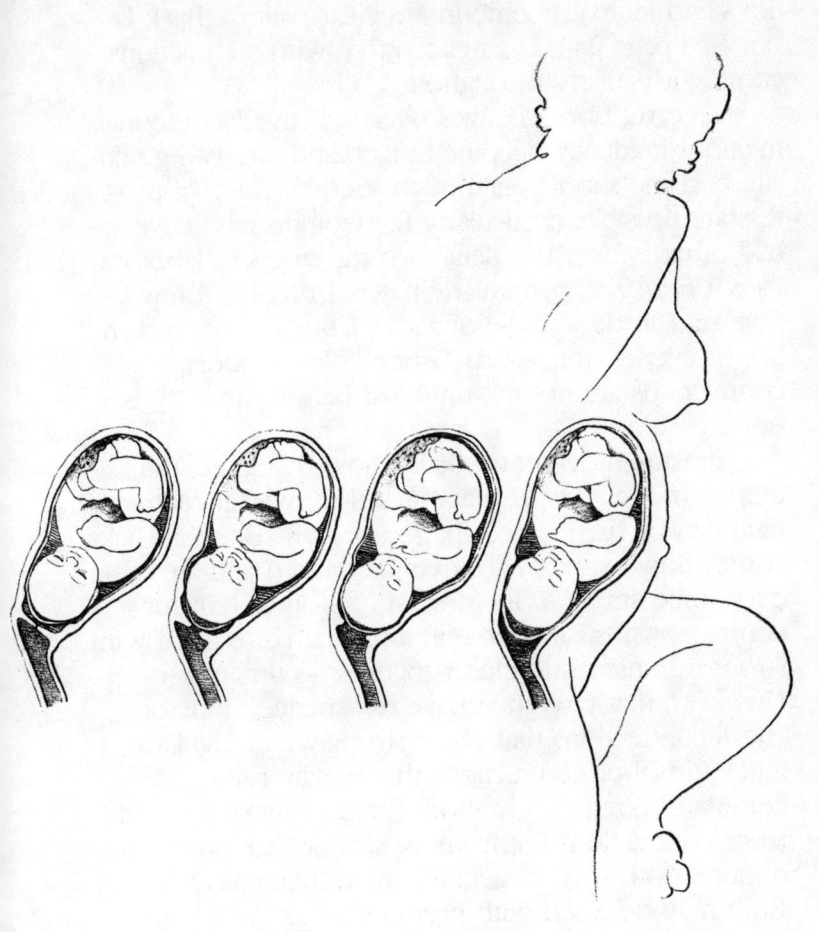

dilating, or opening, until it is fully open and the baby is ready to be born.

CONTRACTIONS

The uterus works in a rhythm, like the heart does—work, rest, work, rest. In almost all labors, contractions and intervals come in a regular pattern. Back labor (see page 244) is an exception, with contractions coming irregularly throughout labor.

As early labor changes over to active labor, contractions gradually become longer, and intervals gradually become shorter—although sudden spurts of progress are possible, particularly for women who have had other babies. For details on the stages of labor, review *Chapter 2*, particularly pages 14 to 19. A few labors start in the middle of active labor with no warm-up, or even in transition. In rare "silent" labors, contractions are not felt until just before the baby is born.

Braxton-Hicks contractions (those that affect the uterus throughout pregnancy) and **early labor contractions** can be hard to tell apart. Typically, Braxton-Hicks contractions come in an irregular pattern and are of an even, mild strength. In contrast, typical early labor contractions usually come in a regular pattern, growing stronger, longer, and closer together as time passes. However, many women have experienced Braxton-Hicks contractions that come strongly and regularly, and early labor contractions that remain mild and come and go unevenly. Both Braxton-Hicks and early labor contractions last from 30 seconds to more than a minute. Both may be accompanied by a backache. Both may be eased with heat (a shower, a bath, a hot-water bottle or heating pad). How can you know the difference? In the very early phase, even your midwife or doctor may not be able to tell if labor has begun. A vaginal exam will show whether the cervix has flattened (effaced) or opened (dilated) more than it had when your partner was last examined. If it has, there is a good chance that this is labor. If not, you and your partner must wait, to see whether the contractions stop or change.

□ □ □

"At first Susan thought it was the sweet and sour pork we had for dinner."

"I felt increasingly strange and crampy and vague urges to stretch my legs and brace myself against something—but cramps as opposed to contractions."

"... had a great urge to sit on the toilet."

"She was feeling dull lower-back pains but she thought she might have caught a draft because she didn't have her back fully covered with blankets."

"... beginning in the lower back, which built to a crescendo and circled to the front, and then eased off."

"It was a tightening feeling, especially grabbing at my lower back. I'm not sure how I knew I was in labor. I just knew. Contractions became regular almost immediately, 5 minutes apart, 30 seconds long, not very strong."

□ □ □

Early labor can be a frustrating time. You don't know when the warm-up contractions (if they *are* warm-up contractions, and not more Braxton-Hicks contractions) will switch over to those of active labor. You may visit the office of your midwife or doctor, or the hospital, several times, only to be sent home because your partner "isn't in labor yet." Your partner may hesitate to lie down to rest because she thinks she may have to get up soon anyway. You may even be wondering if all this might lead up to the sudden appearance of the baby with *you* delivering. For reassurance, read *Born on the Way to the Hospital*, on page 193.

□ □ □

"Labor at home was frustrating because there was no one to tell me how things were progressing."

"After 24 hours my husband and I were in limbo. We gave up cheering on the contractions and I was beginning to feel the whole business was something to be gotten over with."

"When my wife started chest breathing and relaxation, I was on emergency breathing."

□ □ □

It is hard, not knowing exactly what to expect. The only way to cope is to accept what is happening. Concentrate on what you *do* know:

- You do know your partner is having contractions that can be timed.

- You do know how to help her relax with them. (See page 27 for a review of 4-point releasing.)

- You do know how to help her to do slow breathing with them, if she needs to. You can review Slow Breathing on page 30.

- You do know that rest and nourishment (fluids in particular) are important.

- You do know that you can call your midwife or doctor at any time.

- You do know that your partner can be admitted to the hospital if she really prefers to be.

- You do know that the baby will be born eventually, that your waiting will have an end.

While you wait to see whether this is labor, you have a lot with which to work.

WHILE YOU WAIT

Rest. Getting enough rest may be a challenge. Wondering may keep the two of you alert and wakeful. You may become preoccupied as you time contractions. But your partner needs her energy for the labor that is coming, and you need yours to help. So write down contractions for 1 or 2 hours, then put away your paper and pencil until contractions change pace.

Catnaps are valuable. Use them during the day. At night, go to bed. Follow the head-to-toe releasing you have practiced together. When your partner is relaxed enough to rest, lie down and talk yourself through releasing. With luck, you both will sleep.

If contractions keep your partner awake, she may be comfortable working with early labor on her own while you sleep a little. Remember that staying calm and relaxed is her main goal in early labor.

□ □ □

"We had some tea and talked, and finally I made him sleep and I lay down on the sofa with a watch, a pencil and paper, and a book. The sunrise was lovely."

□ □ □

Keep active. When you are not resting, keep yourselves busy. Tensions mount when time hangs heavy on your hands. Avoid hard work, but light activity stimulates labor and encourages a woman's body to function well. At home, your partner can take a shower or a bath if the doctor permits them and if the water bag is unbroken. A slow, gentle massage can be very relaxing. During the day, take a stroll around town. Go for a ride to a beautiful spot. Go to a funny movie. Or you can each continue your own activities, but check with one another once in a while for progress reports and reminders to relax.

□ □ □

"Feeling very proud of ourselves (for no good reason), we went to the Central Park Zoo and had a lovely afternoon."

"We sat in the doctor's office for about half an hour, me breathing away and Bob being very soothing and the whole waiting room staring."

□ □ □

For its calming benefits, keep up the releasing all the time. It is harder to do in labor, and your practicing beforehand will help a lot now.

Remember nutrition. In active labor a woman's digestive system absorbs food and liquids more slowly than usual. This can be a problem if general anesthesia is used at the time of birth. If she vomits before she is fully awake, she can possibly take what has come up from her stomach into her lungs. But in early labor the stomach digests at close to a normal rate. During this time women often are hungry. Find out from your doctor or midwife exactly what your partner may eat. Fluids especially are needed to keep the body working properly.

Foods low in fat and fiber, and foods *not* cooked in fat, are digested most easily. Some of these are:

>Lean fish (perch, flounder, haddock), broiled or baked
>Turkey or chicken without skin, roasted or broiled
>Lowfat and frozen yogurt
>Cottage cheese
>Skim milk
>Toast
>Cooked low-fiber vegetables (carrots, string beans)
>Pureed soups (without cream or whole milk)
>Cooked rice

Remember that your partner should check with the midwife or doctor before eating these or any other foods while she is in labor. Some doctors order clear fluids only. Some of these are:

>Apple, cranberry, or grape juice
>Tea with honey or sugar (no milk)
>Broths (homemade can be salt-free; canned broths usually are quite salty)
>Jello
>Jellied soups
>One glass of wine or hard liquor, if it isn't against your principles—or your doctor's

□ □ □

"The doctor told me to eat breakfast, which I didn't do. This was my first mistake. I was starving by nighttime when I was in active labor."

COACHING

□ □ □

"Claire woke me up to tell me she was ready. I am very proud to say that I was not excited or nervous because I was as ready as could be."

"I said 'That's nice,' rolled back over in bed, and then sat up with a jolt, wondering what to do first."

□ □ □

You can help your partner to keep track of her contractions by timing them with a clock or watch with a second hand. If the pattern is regular, after a while you can predict the start and end of every contraction fairly accurately. If contractions are coming at uneven intervals and lasting for irregular lengths of time, you will have to rely totally on your partner's cleansing breaths to tell you when one starts and stops. By watching your partner's reaction, you may be able to know when a contraction is strongest and how long this peak lasts. When the contraction is over, a reminder to relax helps your partner to let it go.

Especially at the beginning of labor, contractions may seem longer than they are. It can be difficult to tell the difference betwen the contraction itself and the pressure that lingers for several seconds after it is over.

- If you place your hand on your partner's abdomen, you can feel it harden during a contraction. This is easiest with strong contractions. Most laboring women are especially sensitive to touch, and your hand pressure must be very light and gentle. Practice doing this, if your partner is willing, during the last month of pregnancy when Braxton-Hicks contractions come often and usually are not painful. This is a skill that takes a while to learn. In the hospital, nurses, who are experienced, can guide you.

> **Note**: Contractions are timed from the beginning of one to the beginning of the next. For example: a contraction starts at 9 o'clock and ends at 9:01. The next contraction starts at 9:05. Therefore, contractions are coming every 5 minutes (a 1-minute contraction plus a 4-minute interval).

WHEN TO GO TO THE HOSPITAL

Usually, expectant mothers receive instructions from their midwives or doctors about when to contact them if labor seems to have begun. After a telephone conference—and possibly a visit for a vaginal exam—it will be decided whether your partner should go to the hospital now or later. Do not hesitate to call your midwife or doctor to report any signs of labor, day or night—or, if you have already talked, to pass on further developments or to ask questions.

Should your partner feel nervous or uncomfortable at home, even though she has been advised not to come to the hospital yet, you both can make your own decision to go. Just let your midwife or doctor know your plans.

If labor begins strongly and you are hurrying off to the hospital, try to telephone your midwife or doctor before you leave. If you have difficulty getting through, call the hospital. Ask the switchboard operator to tell your midwife or doctor what is happening and that you are coming in. The labor and delivery department will be ready for your arrival.

For the ride to the hospital:

- Keep 1 or 2 large clean towels in your car, starting at the beginning of your partner's ninth month. Tie them up in a plastic bag to keep them clean. A sanitary pad can catch small amounts of fluid leaking from a broken bag of water, but towels are useful for large quantities. The total amount of fluid in the uterus at the end of pregnancy averages $1/2$ to $1 1/2$ pints, but there easily may be more or less. The uterus keeps manufacturing amniotic fluid until the baby is born, so leaking will continue after the bag breaks.

□ □ □

"The amount of fluid was unexpected. I gushed, soaking 6 or 7 pads, and arrived feeling like a 2-year-old who had wet her pants."

□ □ □

- Remember to bring suitcases and labor kit. Take along your partner's hospital insurance card, if she has not already mailed in this information. Bring your own letter or certificate stating that you and your partner have taken a course in education for childbirth.

  Paying attention to your driving and to your partner at the same time is difficult. If you have practiced driving while she relaxes and breathes over the past weeks, both of you will be better able to cope with the real thing. Above all, drive carefully. Stay as calm as you can. Babies rarely are born on the way to the hospital.

□ □ □

"In the car Alice leaned against the window, wet rag on her head and breathed (puff, puff). The car ride calmed her down."

"I remember feeling quite calm and confident that all was happening the way it was supposed to. The ride was nice, snow falling lightly, and just as we crossed the bridge, the sun came through."

"The night we left it was raining and foggy out. Fortunately, a friend rode with us to help Jenny while I concentrated on the road. It's quite difficult to drive and coach at the same time."

"The breathing is a very good aid for ignoring talkative cab drivers."

□ □ □

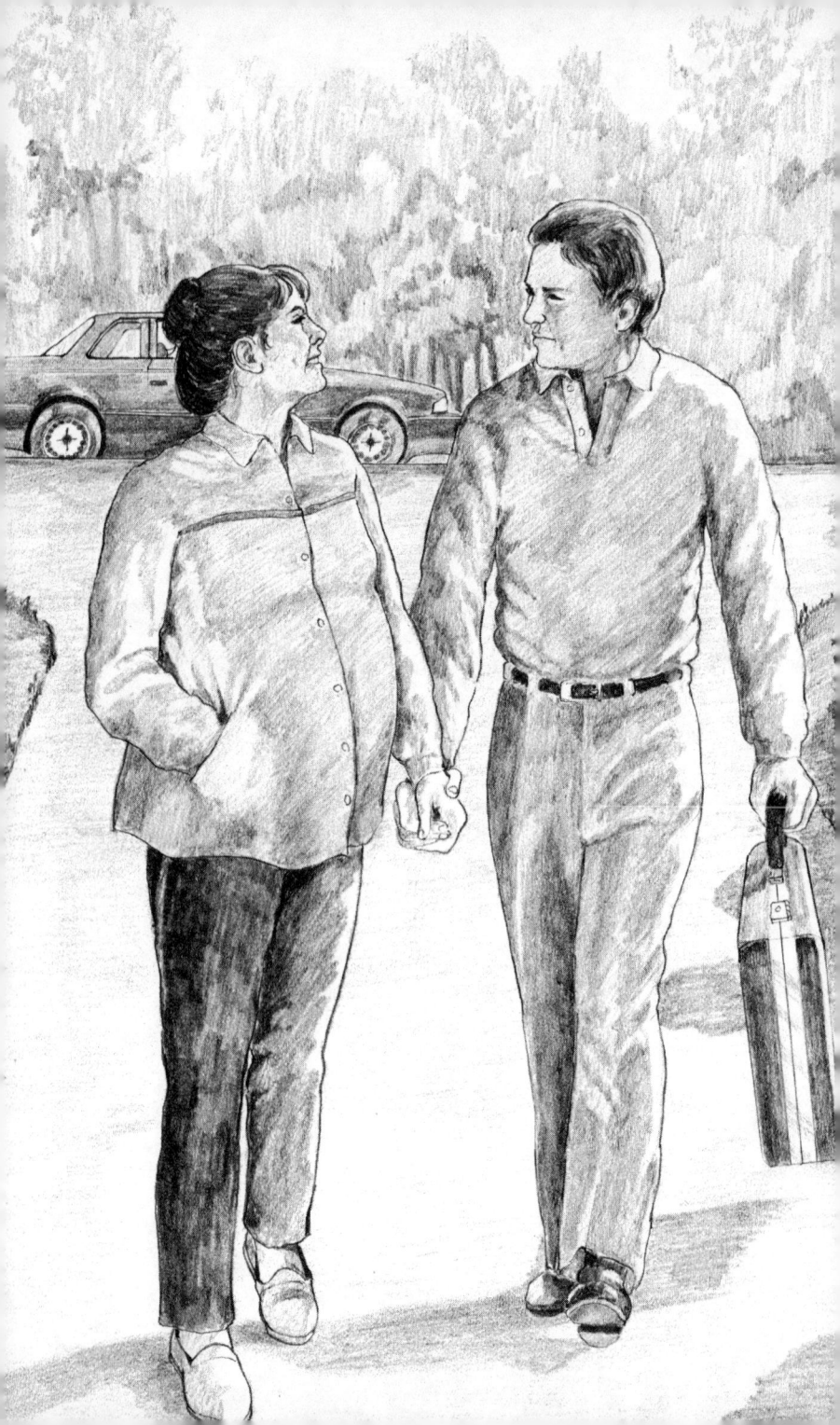

5. Going to the Hospital

Most people go to hospitals to have their babies. Even if your partner and you are going to a birth center, you will want information on hospitals just in case you should be transferred to a traditional hospital labor and delivery unit.

The next few pages will give you a look at birth in a hospital. As you read, check information you especially want to remember so that you can find it quickly and easily when you need it.

BEFORE YOU GO

When a woman gives birth, most of the hospital procedures that affect her directly are ordered by her midwife or doctor. Shaves, enemas, IVs, medications, fetal monitors, and rules about eating or drinking after labor begins are all under his or her direction. An office visit is the time to ask questions and make requests because, if you wait until labor begins, you and your partner, and the midwife or doctor, will be too busy for long discussions.

- At least 3 months before the baby is due, your partner can ask for extra time at one of her appointments so that you can both talk with the midwife or doctor. If there are several in practice together, meet each one at other visits. Sharing a practice does not guarantee that the doctors share similar points of view. Please read more about hospital procedures on page 205.

Some of your requests may be out of your doctor's hands because they are decided by hospital policy. Any procedures called "hospital policy" have been decided by your hospital's board of directors and are described in writing in the hospital policy book. According to the American Hospital Association, patients may read this book if they wish.

- You might ask if your midwife or doctor would mind if you talked with the director of obstetrics and the hospital administrator at your hospital. Write first to both of them, explaining what you would like, then follow through by phoning for an appointment to talk together.

A number of procedures are decided on the spot by hospital nurses, who base their decisions on their experience and judgment, and on your individual circumstances.

- If you and your partner have a request to make during labor, explain to the nurse *what* you want to do and *why* it is important to you. **Sometimes a heartfelt request, politely stated, will go a long way.**

AT THE HOSPITAL

Your first stop in the hospital will be the admissions office. Early in pregnancy, most women receive a preadmission form from their doctors. They fill it in and mail it to the hospital. The admissions office then has most of the information it needs in advance, and your visit there will be short.

- Keep a copy of the completed admission form and bring it with you to the hospital. It will save answering the same questions again, should the original have gone astray (unlikely, but possible). Your partner's insurance information should be on this form. If it is not, she will need her insurance card.

□ □ □

"Marion was preregistered. As a matter of fact I shouted her name to the woman at the desk, told her she was in labor and couldn't wait for her to get off the telephone, and we went straight up to the labor room."

□ □ □

Hospital personnel sometimes forget how hard a woman is working and ask questions or start procedures while she is having a contraction.

- Courteously explain that the contraction will soon be over, and ask if the person would mind waiting until it is. Then turn your attention to your partner, who may have been distracted, and help her to relax and breathe. Make sure she remembers the cleansing breath at the end of the contraction. It will separate her from the contraction when it is over so that she can give her full attention to the question or procedure. Especially in strong labor, women need to center much of their attention inward on themselves. If your partner prefers not to be disturbed and you can supply the answer to the question being asked, this is usually all right with everybody.

A nurse or other hospital attendant will meet you at the admissions office with a wheelchair for your partner. Unless there is a medical reason why she should ride or hospital policy requires it, she may walk to the labor room if she prefers. Pressure from the baby can make sitting uncomfortable.

- After you check with the attendant, ask your partner if she would feel more comfortable walking instead of riding.

□ □ □

"They wouldn't let me walk. I felt fine, but saw no sense in arguing so I rode in the wheelchair."

□ □ □

You may be asked to wait, usually in a father's waiting room, while your partner is admitted as a patient to the hospital. She may find it difficult to be without your support at this time. If you suspect that the baby will be born especially soon, you will have additional reason not to be separated.

- Courteously ask the labor nurse if you may stay with your partner. Explain why it is important to you both.

If you do have to wait awhile in the waiting room, find out how long you can expect to be there. Usually, admission takes about an hour. This time often passes very slowly and you may begin to feel that you have been forgotten, especially if you are not called when you expect to be.

- Ask a nurse or other medical attendant nearby to phone the labor unit and see whether you may come in yet.

□ □ □

"I was left to pace old-style on the sixth floor. This was probably the hardest hour for me. I didn't think I could tolerate the thought of being somewhere else while my child was being born."

"Now that I was nicely settled, I suggested in polite tones that George be allowed up. No one was willing to take the responsibility. I suggested that they call the doctor; he said it was fine. Then it was decided that the doctor had no right to say that. Finally, three hours after my arrival, he came up."

"There is such habit in your body's reactions. When you see your coach, all the practice, all the knowing what she is there for, start to work."

□ □ □

Most hospitals require coaches to wear special clothes, usually in the labor room, always for the birth.

- When your partner goes to be admitted, you can ask the nurse who escorts her for your coaching clothes so that you can change immediately and rejoin her as soon as possible. You will be shown where to change and where to leave your belongings.

- Keep your valuables with you or give them to a labor nurse for safekeeping. Leave what you don't need at home.

Clothing for a coach is either a long-sleeved hospital gown worn over your own clothes, or "scrub clothes" like those worn by midwives, doctors, and nurses—an over-the-head shirt with drawstring pants for men and a simple over-the-head dress for women.

- Wear lightweight clothes. The combination of your own clothing with a hospital gown can be uncomfortably warm.

Admission procedures may include: answering questions, signing forms, a brief physical exam, listening to the baby's heartbeat, the taking of blood and urine samples, an enema, shave, and the use of an IV and fetal monitor. For details on these procedures, see Chapter 10, *What to Expect with Hospital and Medical Procedures,* on page 205).

If your partner has practiced her labor skills on her own (in addition to practicing with you), she will be better prepared to work by herself if you are separated at times like these.

□ □ □

"Reunited, we scuffled into our labor room, a rather drab, uninspiring place. Hospitals should really do more to lighten the place up."

□ □ □

Before you may enter the labor room, some hospitals ask for proof that you have taken a course preparing you for labor and delivery. Childbirth instructors usually give couples a certificate or letter.

- Bring your certificate with you to the hospital.

SETTLING DOWN TO WORK

When you get a chance (probably after all the admission procedures have been completed), here are some things to check in the labor room:

1. If you and your partner have a special request list, give it to the medical attendant and ask that it be attached to your partner's chart. Keep a copy to show the midwife or doctor when she or he arrives, just as a reminder of your previous conversations.

2. Quiet surroundings with indirect lighting will make working with labor easier.

   - Try substituting a floor lamp or a wall light for an overhead light. If there are overhead lights only, perhaps the one directly over your partner's bed can be shut off. Perhaps a night light would be adequate. Or is there a window that admits enough daylight?

   - You may decide to ask politely for quiet if there is a lot of talking and action directly around you.

> **If things that make you uncomfortable cannot be changed,** you are better off to concentrate on what *is* working for you instead of on what isn't. Put your energy into being together and using your labor skills and teamwork.

3. Find out how to raise and lower the entire bed. Back rubs are easier for you to do with the mattress up at the level of your waist. Your partner can climb in and out more comfortably when the bed is close to the floor.

4. Find out how to raise the head of the bed so that your partner may sit up, if she wants to, with full

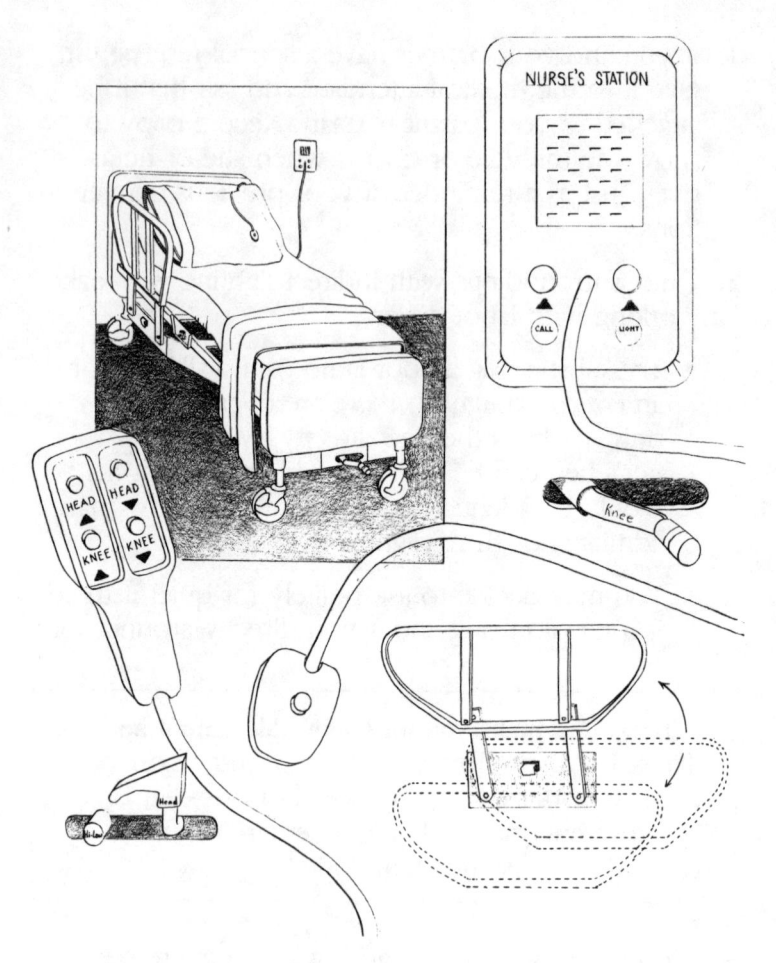

Bed controls and call buttons

support for her back. And find out how to raise the mattress under her knees for a more comfortable position. Legs can relax best when the joints are slightly bent. (Sometimes pillows or mattresses under the knees are not permitted. The concern is that pressure there over a long period of time may cause circulation problems. As with anything that is sometimes allowed and sometimes not, ask before you assume that the answer is "no" for you.)

5. Find out where supplies are kept. For example, you may need:

- Extra pillows or pillow cases. If you brought in extra pillows from home, these should be covered with plastic and labeled with your name.

- Absorbent pads (for under your partner) and waste basket (for those that are used).

- Towels and washcloths. At least two should be available for sponge baths, back compresses, and wetting dry lips and mouth.

- Basins, to hold water for compresses and bathing.

- Hot and cold running water, for compresses.

- Emesis basin, for throwing up.

- Ice chips, for sucking (if it is allowed), for cold water compresses, and for bathing.

- Drinking water and paper cups, and the soda machine for ginger ale, if liquids are allowed and you did not bring your own.

- Coaches' bathroom.

- Call bell, for calling the nurse if she is out of the room and you need her.

- A chair for you to sit in.

WORKING WITH DOCTORS AND NURSES

It often comes as a surprise to find that your doctor and perhaps your midwife will not be with you constantly during labor, even though he or she may be somewhere in the hospital. The nurse keeps track of labor and passes on reports regularly. She herself may not be with you at all times either. Often this is because she is busy, but she also may feel that you prefer privacy.

You may find that you need advice about coaching or want something explained.

- Use your call bell or go in search of the nurse—she will be nearby. If you prefer not to leave your partner, don't hesitate to shout "NURSE!"

□ □ □

"Everything we requested from the hospital staff was agreed to, BUT you must ask. If you ask for nothing, you get nothing."

"I was very fortunate that the hospital staff respected my wishes and cooperated with me to the best of their ability. This is extremely important. Someone who treats you like a lunatic can be most disconcerting."

□ □ □

Sometimes we worry that our questions are silly or that we are being a nuisance when we ask them. All questions need answers. Getting the facts helps you to cope. If there is something you want to know, ask. If you want to talk with the doctor, simply say so. He can be paged and, if he is not in the hospital, he is only a phone call away.

GETTING WHAT YOU WANT

Advance planning—becoming informed, talking with your midwife or doctor, and your hospital—is the key to a happy hospital experience. Nevertheless, you may run into a procedure or an attitude that is not in keeping with your expectations or beliefs. Many people are a little intimidated around hospitals, and you and your partner are particularly vulnerable because so much of your energy is needed for coping with labor. These suggestions may help toward making sure you are seen and heard, while you keep on friendly working terms with the staff.

1. Be sure that you yourself clearly understand what you want.

2. Believe in your point of view. State it with confidence. Look directly into the eyes of the person to whom you are speaking. You need not be apologetic.

3. Say *what* you want, and *why*. Give the reasons for your request.

4. Come to the point briefly and directly.

5. State your wish positively. Focus on what you want, instead of what you don't want. For example, try "My partner is having trouble concentrating. I think quiet would help. Would you talk outside the room?" instead of "Your talking is annoying my partner."

6. Honey works better than vinegar. Speak quietly, pleasantly, courteously. Offer requests rather than

demands. "May we have some privacy?" rather than "These student nurses have to leave our room!"

7. Expect the best. It is much harder to get what you want when you have a chip on your shoulder. "We would like to try this pushing method for a few contractions to see how it goes," rather than "This is how we learned it, and this is how we'll do it!"

8. See yourself as enlisting the aid of a staff person to achieve what you want. A friendly nurse can be an ally and mediator when you have difficulty talking with someone, even if that person happens to be your own doctor or midwife.

9. Use a sense of humor when it suits the moment.

10. Midwives, doctors, and staff are human beings and, like anyone else, appreciate being appreciated—with a smile, a compliment, a thank you.

11. You may become angry. Everyone has the right to feel anger, and you can decide whether or not you want to express it. Be as calm as you can be. Be direct.

12. Being angry may make you nervous. You may decide to speak up in spite of feeling nervous. Try a deep, slow, quiet breath along with relaxing from head to toe.

13. Your midwife's or doctor's word—by telephone or in person—can straighten out a difficult situation.

14. Should you and your midwife or doctor have a completely irreconcilable difference of opinion, you always have the option of requesting a second opinion from another midwife or obstetrician.

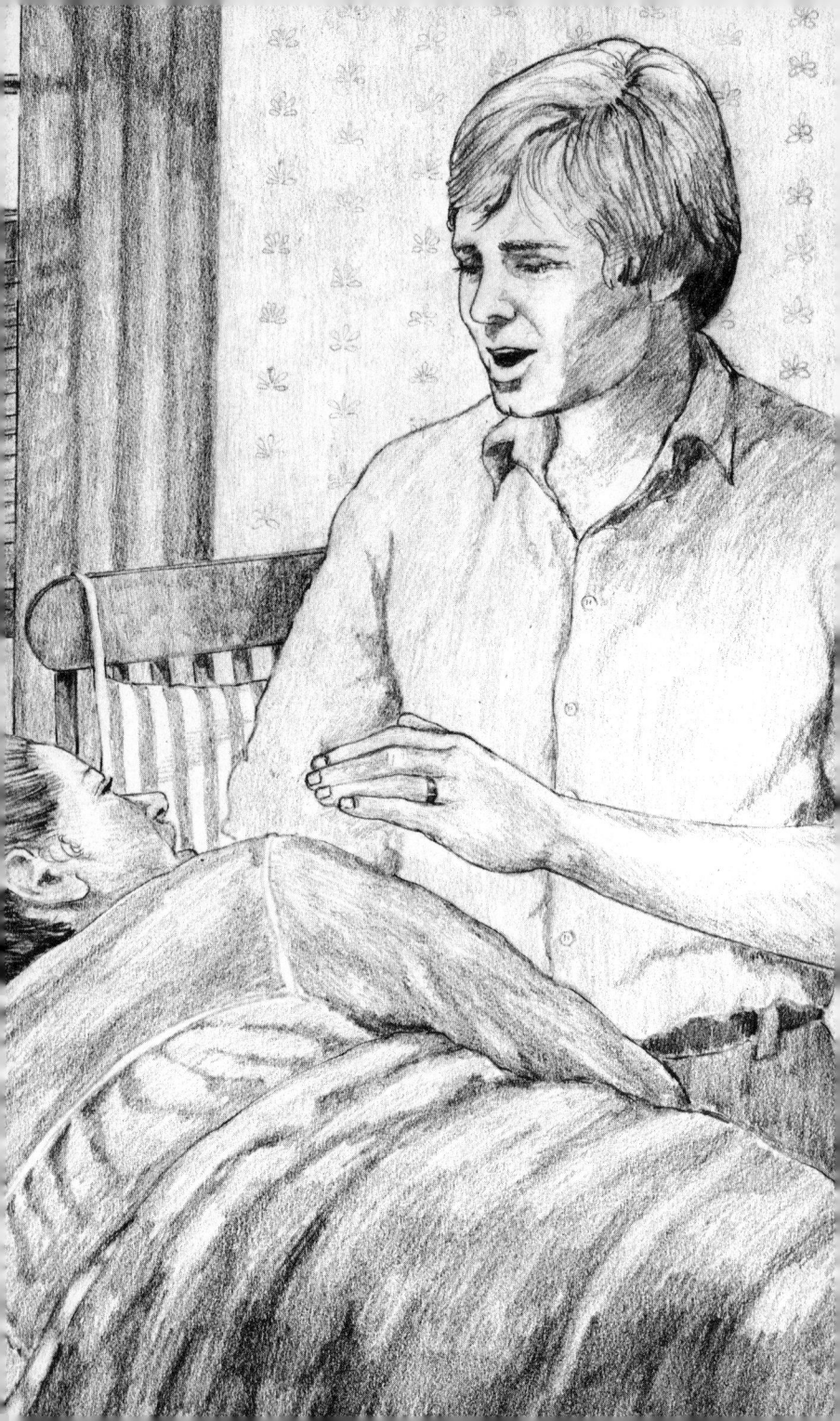

6. The Coach's Skills (General Principles)

This is the first of three chapters on the nitty-gritty of coaching for labor. The preliminaries are over. There you are in the hospital and this is the real thing. This chapter deals with the general principles that underlie your role as coach. Chapter 7 gives step-by-step details for the stages of labor. In Chapter 8 you learn what to expect once the baby arrives. At the end of each chapter is an easy-to-follow summary for quick reference.

By now you are familiar with the skills your partner will use to help herself throughout labor and—provided you are well practiced—you can guide her in their use.

But labor is more than a physical process. How do you communicate with someone who, because she is hard at work, seems to pay no attention to you at times? How does she feel, and what does she need to cope with those feelings beyond knowing how to relax, breathe, and push? What about simple physical comfort? What *really* works to boost the confidence of a woman in labor? What are the tricks to hanging in there yourself, when you are bored and tired?

Most of the answers are common sense, geared to labor. These pointers will help to round out your effectiveness as coach.

KNOWLEDGE

To take part in a labor and delivery, you must have information about how a woman's body gives birth, about the attitudes of your midwife or doctor, about hospital routines. Then, instead of feeling like an ignorant bystander, you will have a basic picture of what the medical personnel are discussing, and of the many natural processes that might otherwise seem to you strange or abnormal.

When you are informed, variations from a textbook labor—to be expected in all labors—are more easily understood and dealt with.

The knowledge you will use includes an understanding of your partner's relaxing, breathing, and pushing skills (Chapter 3). Your own coaching skills, described in these chapters, will help you to feel confident in passing along realistic and workable reminders, demonstrations, explanations, guidance.

WORKING WITH THE MOMENT

Labor is definitely a waiting game. As a coach you will discover that one very useful skill is knowing *how* to wait. It can be difficult. You are unable to affect the pace of labor. As you wait for time to pass, you will not even know how many hours to plan on. You are confined to a limited space. You are focused on one basic task that requires constant concentration while, to some degree, you must feel your way along. Several hours may pass during which little happens to reassure you that progress is being made. It is understandable that you may become restless, nervous, possibly bored—and that your responses become automatic rather than planned.

"During the whole thing, time seemed to drag, but looking back I guess it flew."

◻ ◻ ◻

The best way for you as coach to get through labor and to absorb the full experience, is to try not to wish time away, but rather to involve yourself with what is happening at the moment. When this works, it is like wrapping a cocoon of calmness around yourself and your partner in which you work together moment by moment. In most cases, a woman's body will do its own thing in its own time. In the meantime, focus directly on the present.

OBSERVING

Use your eyes. Watch your partner carefully, from head to toe. What you learn by observing gives you clues as to her needs. Does she look comfortable? Do you see tension anywhere? Is her deep breathing slow, and her rapid breathing shallow? What is her mood?

She may look obviously uncomfortable to you, although she may not realize it herself because she is so absorbed in labor. You may spot tension in a frown, hunched shoulders, clenched hands. You may notice that breathing is more rapid and less relaxed than it was in practice. Often, you can keep little problems from becoming big ones by heading off trouble before it gets a toehold.

ENCOURAGEMENT

Encouragement keeps your partner going. It strengthens her belief in herself. This holds true at all times during labor. For a woman in labor, loneliness and fear of the unknown are tough enemies. There is no way to measure the value of yourself, a loving, caring friend at her side. Your presence is, in itself, reassuring.

- Offer support, not criticism. Give her credit for what she can do, letting her know that her efforts are recognized. This makes her feel less alone and more confident.

□ □ □

"He talked the entire time, telling me how much he loved me and how great I was doing. At this state, I thought him a terrific liar (I was feeling miserable)."

"I spent very little time talking (unlike in practice) and much more time actually breathing with her, trying to pace her. My wife never panicked but came close a few times. I just kept breathing with her and held her tightly."

"We didn't speak a lot but he was just there by my side the whole time, and it was important to me to see him acting normally, unafraid (though tired) and just being with me."

□ □ □

Praise her often and at any time. She gains confidence from knowing that her efforts are appreciated. As a coach, you may be so busy offering reminders and correcting mistakes that you forget to mention those things that are going well.

- Specific praise is more effective than generalities. A laboring woman may interpret praise as a kind of white lie to cheer her up. A specific comment is more believable. For example, tell your partner, "You are relaxing your shoulders beautifully" rather than, "You are doing very well." Being specific also helps to strengthen her focus on the labor skills that are designed to help her.

- Be honest. Don't promise what you cannot deliver. Statements like "This won't hurt. This won't take long. Labor will last another hour. This contraction has only 15 more seconds to go" are guesses because you cannot know for sure. Ultimately such statements can be disappointing. If your truthful answer to a question is "I don't know," it is probably best to say so. It helps your partner to be able to depend on your answer—even if it is not the one she wants.

- It is most useful to work totally in the present, contraction by contraction, rest period by rest period. Think of a bicyclist, tired and hot, sore, looking down miles of a long road and wondering how she can possibly make it to the end. If she aims for a landmark close at hand, however, she knows that she can reach her goal. Sign post by sign post, she will find herself at the end of the road, eventually.

TOUCHING

Touch is a tremendously important tool to use in helping your partner through labor.

Touch is a reminder to let go of tension. Even though you *tell* your partner that she needs to relax a certain part of her body (her shoulders, for example), she may not realize that she is tense there until you touch that spot.

Touch is also a way of signaling your partner to pay attention to you. For example, when you help her through a difficult contraction by breathing along with her, you can remind her to concentrate on your teamwork, more than on the contraction, by touching her hand or shoulder.

Stroking or massage can be soothing. Abdominal stroking feels good and can ease pain. Back rubs or back pressure (see page 246) can ease back or at least help to make it tolerable.

Different ways of touching are effective for different people. Sometimes people hesitate to touch others, associating touch with sexuality. It may help to recognize that here it is a form of silent communication, expressing comfort, reassurance, and caring at a time when speech may be inadequate or annoying. Have confidence. Ask yourself how you might like to be touched.

- Smooth tension away by stroking your partner gently in one direction, *away* from her body. This tends to draw tension out of her body. For example, stroke down her arm toward her fingertips, or down her thighs toward her knees. Or gently rest your hand on a tense body part and suggest that she imagine the warmth of your hand drawing the tension out of her body like a magnet. You probably will create some of your own techniques to ease your partner's tension.

□ □ □

"The leg pain was the most uncomfortable part of every contraction. My husband helped me tremendously by rubbing my legs."

"There was no way Betsey wanted to be touched at all and therefore my efforts were confined to breathing with and talking to her. The no-touch reaction did not surprise me, for I know that in similar moments of effort and stress I have not wanted any interference with my concentration."

> **Note**: During hard work in labor—in transition, for example—some mothers find it very annoying to be touched, and may say so abruptly. Understand that it is the demands of labor, and not you, that might cause your partner to be super-sensitive. If she does not want to be touched, then you can rely on talking.

□ □ □

"Her belly was too sore to be rubbed, but it was cold, so I rested my hands on her abdomen to warm it."

□ □ □

TALKING (AND LISTENING, AND SILENCE)

Communicating in labor is different from the kind of everyday communication we often take for granted. Because so much of a mother's attention is focused on herself, especially during contractions, communication is simpler, more direct, centered around the mother's needs.

A quiet tone creates calm.

A firm tone can strengthen her resolve to stay in control when pain and fatigue may tempt her to give up. Occasionally you may need to raise your voice to get her attention.

Your partner may be too involved with her feelings and her work to volunteer comments or requests, and it is important that you recognize this.

- Wait for intervals between contractions to ask questions that need answers, to suggest changes, or to review techniques. This is when your partner can talk with you.

- Check with your partner from time to time, to see if your efforts to help her are working. Would she prefer that you do what you are doing differently, or that you change to something else?
- Ask your partner occasionally whether she needs anything. You cannot assume that she will tell you.
- During contractions, make only comments that will help her as she works. Recognize that, in order to work well, she must concentrate on one thing only—coping with the contraction. You can support her effort by concentrating on the same thing.

□ □ □

"My concentration was absolute. I didn't want to be spoken to during a contraction, and was almost in a trance-like state in between."

□ □ □

Try to direct whatever you say to the basic goal of understanding, and creating a working link among everyone who shares the experience of helping your partner through labor and birth. Use simple words to express exactly what you mean, especially to your partner. Use few words, to get your message across without complication.

Listening is the flip side of talking, and is just as important. When your partner has something to tell you, *listen*. Put yourself on her wavelength, because she can't adjust to yours while she is working in labor. Consider what she says as fact, not hysteria. A woman in labor may not be a medical expert, but often she knows intuitively what is happening with her body.

Silence, the opposite of talk, has value too. The noise of voices, even yours, may annoy your partner to the point where she cannot concentrate. She may say so bluntly, either voluntarily or when you ask.

Some women need total quiet in order to concentrate fully. This ideal situation is hard to achieve in a hospital, but you can ask the staff to help your partner by talking outside your room.

Occasionally another woman in labor, frightened and unhappy, may make a lot of noise. This can become distracting and worrying for your partner, who will start to wonder when it will be her turn to lose control.

- Remind her that she has her labor skills and that she also has you, her coach, to keep her going.

- During contractions, and intervals as well, work closely with your partner, encouraging her to concentrate as totally as possible on the skills she is using.

▫ ▫ ▫

"It never crossed my mind that I would hear other women in labor like that. I guess I thought everyone would have taken Lamaze courses."

▫ ▫ ▫

BEING THE GO-BETWEEN

You may be the go-between for your partner and the medical attendants.

- If explanations by the staff are hard to understand, find out what is meant and pass along the information to your partner in brief, simple terms.

- Ask hospital staff to wait until a contraction is finished before asking questions or doing procedures. One exception might be a vaginal exam; for details, see page 206.

For a laboring woman, sensitive to everything, environment is very important. It will help if you are alert to your surroundings and find out from your partner what puts her at ease. For example, one woman may feel excluded and forgotten when coach and doctor converse about everyday matters. Another may feel that the same chat keeps her company without demanding her response.

Although the basic goals for breathing and pushing skills agree, the techniques themselves vary a little. It can be confusing if the suggestions of the staff differ from your particular approach.

- An explanation from you to the staff helps.

The staff also may have some useful tips. If their suggestions fit in with what you and your partner are trying to achieve, you might give them a try.

- You may decide to adopt the new idea, stick with your own approach, or blend the two, depending on which works best.

Remember that the medical staff—nurses, midwives, doctors—are your teammates, not your critics. Their first concern is the physical safety of your partner, while yours is helping her to cope with labor. If some of your viewpoints are different, you may feel that you cannot work together. However, usually you can. Unless your ideas are unsafe for your partner or the baby, a courteous explanation often will win cooperation. If you meet resistance, and you are fully clear on the issue, you may need to persist to make your point. Please read page 97 for more suggestions on being assertive.

> **Remember**: Good humor, courtesy, and a word or two of explanation often get the point across.

GIVING DIRECTIONS

The simpler the directions, the easier they are to follow. A reminder to "remember when you push, you must relax your bottom and keep your back rounded, and bring your head forward; use your abdominal muscles, and keep your mouth open," is confusing instead of helpful because it is long-winded and too complicated. Offer one simple suggestion at a time, wait until she responds, then offer the next. "Now relax your bottom. [pause] Good. Now round your back. [pause] Very good. Now bring your head forward..." and so on.

Keep your voice gentle and calm. At the same time, use a tone of quiet authority.

Use as few words as possible, and express exactly what you mean. Your partner's attention centers more and more on herself as labor becomes more active, so that she has little attention to spare, to figure out your meaning if you are vague.

The order of directions can be important. When you say "relax your *bottom*, keep your *back* rounded, bring your *head* forward, use your *abdominal* muscles, keep your *mouth* open" you name body parts at random, and confusingly. Follow the line of her body to make more sense—head, mouth, back, abdomen, bottom.

Directions need to be positive. If you say "Don't breathe so fast" to your partner, it only discourages her by telling her she is breathing "wrong." It tells her what *not* to do, but leaves her without direction. Try "You are breathing too fast. Breathe more slowly, like this. (demonstrate) Let's try it together." If you must start a sentence with "don't," follow it immediately with a statement of what *should* be done.

Directions should be specific. If you say "You need to relax more," the direction is too general to be of much help. She is too preoccupied with what she is doing to translate this message into a usable form. Say exactly what you mean. Try "release your head/neck/shoulders." Wait until she responds, then go on to the next specific step.

Demonstrate your suggestions. Especially when your partner is working very hard and can spare only a little attention, it may be easiest for her to understand you if she watches and copies your actions. "Now you must stop pushing. Use your pant-blow breathing. Like this. Watch me. Breathe with me...."

WATCHING OUT FOR HER COMFORT

Something unexpected happens when a mother-to-be enters a hospital to have a baby. Because she is excited and usually a little nervous, and because the surroundings are unfamiliar, she forgets about making herself comfortable, and she loses her nerve about asking questions. As coach, you can fill in the blanks. Reassured that the extras are being taken care of by you, your partner is free to concentrate fully on working with her labor.

Nurses often take over many of the tasks of making mothers comfortable, because your main concern is to help your partner work with her contractions. But there are simple ways to help her to relax, to feel cared for, and to be more comfortable. Knowing about them, you might choose to do them yourself, especially if the staff is very busy.

□ □ □

"Those little niceties that seemed inconsequential during class attained terrific importance during labor."

□ □ □

A woman may find it difficult to protest when her position is uncomfortable, while she is in labor and in unfamiliar surroundings.

- Find out at what angle your partner would like her bed to be. Does she need pillows for support, and where does she want them? Would she prefer to try another position, in bed or out of bed?

Mothers often do not feel pressure from a full bladder because their attention is taken up by the pressure of the contracting uterus. A full bladder, however, keeps the baby from moving down into the pelvis during labor.

- Every hour or so, ask your partner if she needs to empty her bladder.

- While it is usually all right to go to the bathroom rather than using the bedpan, check with the nurse first. You can also help with slippers and something around your partner's shoulders to keep her warm, as well as by holding her hospital gown closed behind her. These little things that we do automatically for ourselves can seem like gigantic tasks to a mother in labor.

- So that your partner can get out of her high hospital bed with the least effort, it must be lowered close to the floor. A handle or button to raise or lower the bed is usually found at the foot of the bed. If the bed is not adjustable, there should be a stool nearby.

- If your partner has an IV running, ask the nurse for a pole on which to hang the bottle. The pole then can be pushed across the floor as you walk along.

- Stay with your partner in the bathroom if she needs you.

- If she is confined to bed and must use a bedpan, she will be more comfortable if she sits on it at the edge of her bed with her legs over the side and her feet resting on a chair.

If your partner's mouth is dry, offer a sip of water or other clear fluids if her doctor permits this. If she may not have fluids, offer a lick of a sour lollipop or a fresh lemon, or some chips of ice to suck on (if ice is permitted, the nurse will tell you where to find it).

- To keep her body fluids at a healthy level, sips of fluid are important if she does not have an IV running.

- The lollipop may be kept in a glass of ice water to keep it more refreshing. Sometimes the sugar in candy adds to thirst instead of relieving it. Ask her if this is happening.

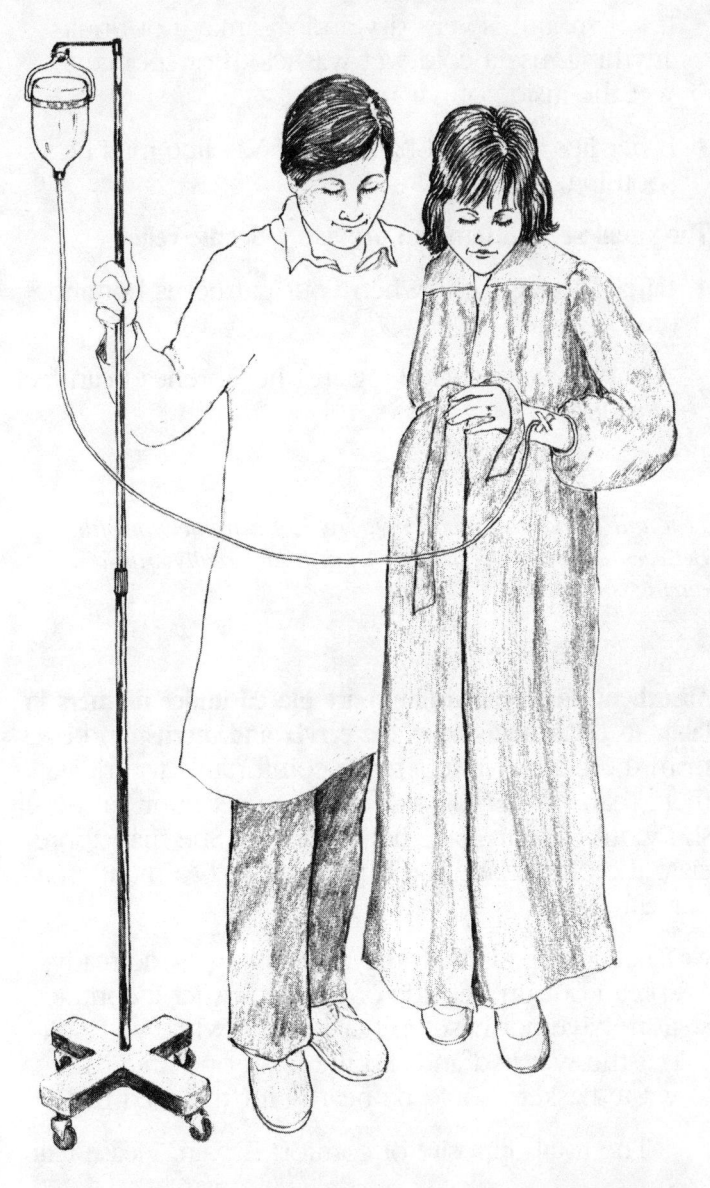

Walking, with a travelling IV pole

- If her mouth is very dry and she may not drink anything, use a cold wet washcloth or sponge to wet the inside of her mouth.

- If her lips are dry, Chapstick or Vaseline may be soothing.

The smallest attention can provide welcome relief.

- Offer sponge baths when your partner is hot and tired.

- A cold, wet washcloth against her forehead can feel wonderful.

▫ ▫ ▫

"I found the washcloth on my forehead extremely helpful. Between contractions I didn't want it, but really craved it during contractions."

▫ ▫ ▫

Absorbent pads (called Chux) are placed under mothers in labor to catch fluids from the cervix and uterus, and even from the bladder if it is more comfortable to urinate there than on the toilet or bedpan. Ask your partner if she would like to have hers changed. She may appreciate the offer if she is too preoccupied to mention it herself.

- To change pads with the least fuss, get one ready, spread out on the side of the bed. After a contraction, have her raise up her bottom while you pull out the wet pad and slip the fresh one under her. A waste basket should be nearby for the used pad.

The total opposite of comfort is pain. Please read

Coping with Pain on page 187), and the details on back labor, on page 244.

HELPING YOURSELF

It can be easy to overlook your own needs while your partner is the center of attention. Don't neglect yourself. You will be in better shape to coach effectively, and to gain the most from your experience, if you are not exhausted and irritable.

Well before the due date, you may find it very helpful to ask another person to assist you and your partner in labor, someone who has attended many births and has coaching experience plus familiarity with hospital routine. This might be a teacher of childbirth classes or a labor and delivery nurse, someone whom both you and your partner trust and like. If the idea appeals to you, ask your childbirth teacher for names of available people. Your midwife, doctor, or your hospital's maternity nurses may have suggestions, too.

□ □ □

"She never once broke down in front of me though she was just as discouraged as I was at times. She would leave the room to get her head together, then come back in and start all over again, telling me to concentrate on my breathing and relax. She would remind me why I was going through it all."

□ □ □

Practice 4-point releasing for yourself every day, starting several weeks before labor is due to begin. Your mind feels calmer when you can let go of physical tension.

Relaxing, which is a skill, must be learned in advance to use when you need it—in labor or any other time.

During labor, take a break from time to time. Ease the strain if you are working hard, or if it is difficult for you to sit still or to be in one place for long stretches of time. A few minutes to yourself can restore your energy. Walk around, or run in place. Stretch. Take several slow, deep breaths.

You may have to balance your needs against those of your partner. Especially if she is having strong contractions and working hard to stay in control, she should not be left by herself.

- Ask a nurse to take your place while you are away. If the nurse cannot come right away, find out when she can and try to stick it out until she arrives.

- If time passes and she still has not arrived, don't hesitate to ask her again.

Eat! Feeling lightheaded, shaky, or grumpy because you are hungry will interfere with your ability to help your partner.

- Hospital snack bars and cafeterias are usually a long way from the labor room. The hour it may take for a meal may be more time than your partner feels she can be without you. At night, dining rooms often are closed. Coffee offered by the nurses and candy from vending machines are not adequate nourishment, so bring your own food from home. Cheese, fruit, raw vegetables, cans of juice, and thermoses of soup are easy to pop into a bag as you leave for the hospital.

Hospital policy may not permit you to eat in the labor room. If there are no such regulations, check with your partner before eating in front of her. The sight and smell of food may make your partner hungry in early labor—unfair, if she is forbidden by her doctor to eat—or nauseated in active labor. You can always step just outside or go to the fathers' waiting room.

- Women in labor are very sensitive to smells. Coffee, garlic, cigarette breath are hard to take. Supply yourself with mints, gum, or mouthwash.

□ □ □

"The one thing we forgot to bring was a snack for the coach. After 9 hours of no food in the labor room, I began to feel faint. Ellie didn't want me to leave, so we agreed that I would run down to the machine in the lobby and get back in the 4 minutes between contractions. A candy bar kept me going for 5 more hours."

□ □ □

If your partner is in active labor and you feel the need for sleep, there are ways to nap without leaving her.

- You may be able to relax together on a couch or bed. Or you can pull your chair up so that you are facing your partner's bed. Between contractions, put your arms on the mattress, rest your head on them, and doze off. Use your head-to-toe relaxing. When a contraction starts, her cleansing breath may wake you or she can touch your arm. You can work with her and then rest again.

- When you have to work straight through and have no time for any sleep, 4-point releasing will help you to keep from getting tense and to conserve your energy.

□ □ □

"He would fall asleep and I would have to hit him or yell at him so he could wake up and rub my back during a contraction."

□ □ □

Go to the bathroom when you need to. You can work better if you are comfortable. Usually, the bathrooms attached to labor or birthing rooms are reserved for mothers. Find out from the nurse which bathroom you may use. Ask her to fill in for you while you are away.

Get assistance for yourself if you need it. Ask questions, ask for advice, ask for help. Medical attendants will be close by.

- Except to do routine exams, medical attendants often stay away from a laboring couple because they respect your privacy. Unless they are very busy, they usually are glad to keep you company or help with coaching. If, on the other hand, they are around too much, it is easy to ask "Could we be alone for awhile?"

□ □ □

"We were on our own for a long time. I had imagined that there would be a nurse or someone with us all the time and if her breathing wasn't right, a nurse could tell her how to correct it. That was when I was really glad we had our training."

Believe in yourself. Some of the time you will know exactly what to do, some of the time you will be guessing. Trial and error is a necessary part of any team work. When you get an idea, tell your partner (between contractions) what you plan to try. Ask her what she thinks. She may accept or veto the idea. If she is uncertain, try it out. When an idea doesn't work, regard it as a step in learning rather than feeling that you have failed. Sometimes the process of elimination is the only way you both can figure out what is useful and what isn't. And an idea that is not effective now may be just the thing later.

Try to keep your ego out of coaching. Don't take criticism personally. Remember that it is the constant hard work that can cause your partner to be supersensitive and sometimes irritable.

- Sometimes a hospital staff member will get better results than you do. For your partner, this person is the authority and consequently carries a lot of weight. Remember that you and the hospital staff make up a team, each of you bringing your own irreplaceable skills, to help your partner through labor in the best possible way. There is no way that a medical attendant can replace you as a loving, caring friend.

□ □ □

"I had been trying, not very successfully, to get her to relax for over an hour. Then the doctor walked in and said casually 'why don't you relax?' and she went limp."

"I would not listen to the doctor and nurses, only to Dan, and he repeated everything they said."

"Dr. F. at that time was like a drill sergeant, just what I needed. My husband could not act that stern with me after going through all day and evening."

"The nurse gently and tactfully helped me with my responsibilities. During the pushing hours when Pam and I were both exhausted, she took over the coaching."

□ □ □

Quick Coaching Guide (General Principles)

Know what to expect.

- Know the mother's labor skills (see Chapter 3, page 21).
- Know labor and hospital routines.

Know how to wait.

- Keep involved in the labor.
- Focus on the present, instead of worrying about past and future.
- Meet your own needs.

To keep your partner going:

- Encourage her. Praise her. Point out what she does well.
- Watch her to help head off little problems before they become big problems.
- Be honest. Don't promise what you can't deliver, but be optimistic.
- Work with contractions, one at a time. Remain flexible and inventive. Remember, trial and error is realistic.

To communicate:

- Be direct. Keep it simple. Keep it short.
- Wait for intervals between contractions to ask questions that need answers.
- During contractions, make supportive comments.
- Find out if your partner has requests or needs that are not being met.
- Listen carefully.
- Regard the medical staff as teammates.
- Act as go-between.
- Remember the value of silence.

To give directions:

- Use few and simple words.
- Use a calm, gently authoritative voice.
- Use touch, when necessary, to command attention.
- Be specific.
- Be positive ("do") instead of negative ("don't").
- Demonstrate your suggestions.

To ensure your partner's comfort:

- Check her position.
- Remind her to empty her bladder every 1 or 2 hours.
- If her mouth is dry, offer fluids, ice chips, sour lollipops, lemon wedges,—if these are allowed—Vaseline, Chapstick

- Offer sponge baths.
- Use powder or cornstarch for massages.

To relieve tension:

- Remind her of 4-point releasing.
- Stroke her limbs in one direction, away from her body.
- Use abdominal stroking, back pressure, massage, when they feel good to your partner.
- Be sure her position is as comfortable as possible.

To help yourself:

- Relax with 4-point releasing.
- Take a break now and then.
- Eat—remembering to be considerate of your partner's heightened sensitivities during labor.
- Go to the bathroom.
- Ask the staff to help you when necessary.
- Believe in yourself.

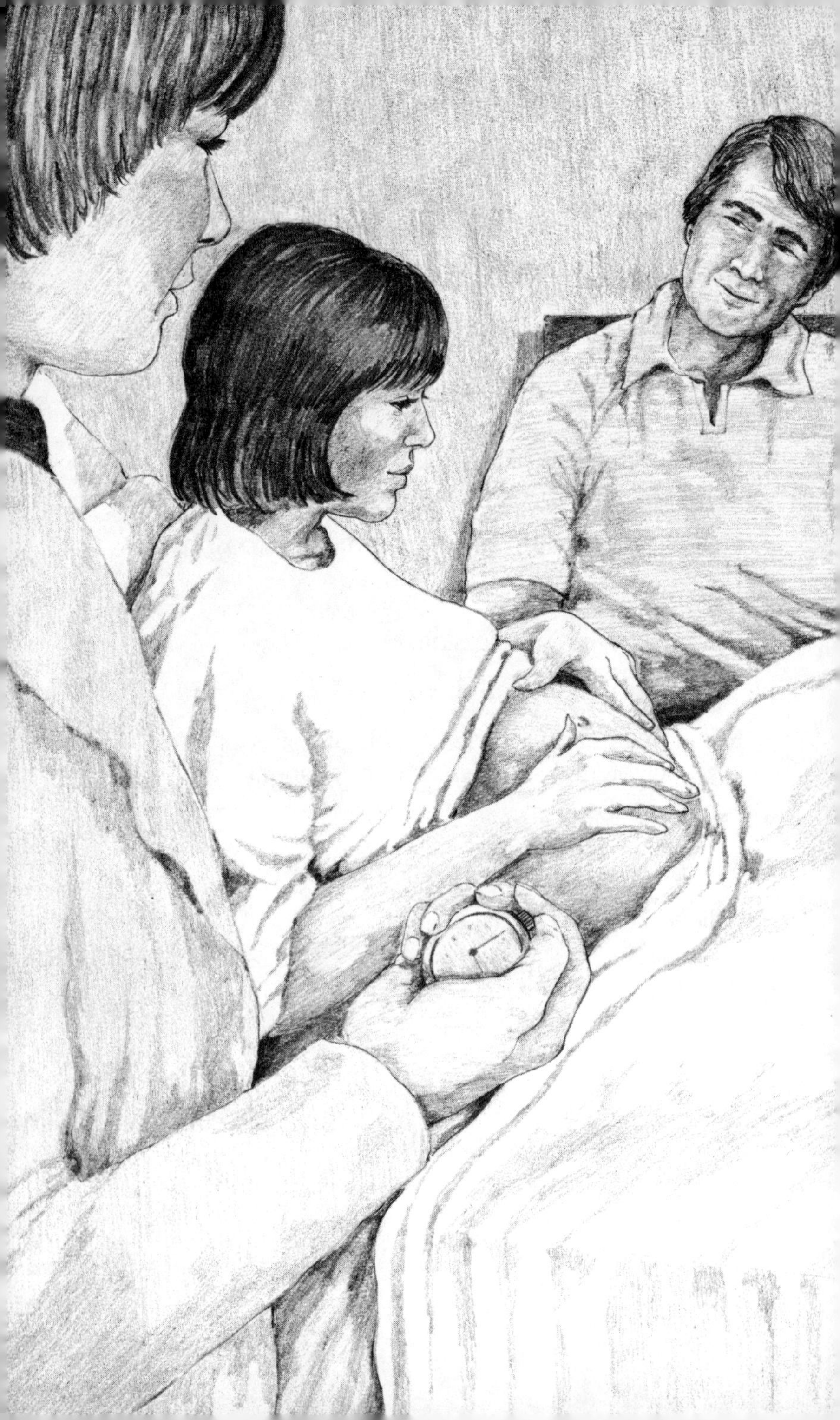

7. The Coach's Skills (The Stages of Labor)

Here is a step-by-step look at labor, from the early warm-up at home, through active labor and birth in the hospital. Reading this will be a little like dress rehearsal for you, except that all the action is on paper. Your script is different from a play script, however. In a play the lines and the action are preset. Every labor, is different. You and your partner will adapt what you know to your individual experience. Understanding the overall picture gives you a foundation from which to respond.

EARLY LABOR (BEGINNING OF STAGE 1)

Usually, early labor is most happily spent outside the hospital (see also Chapter 4: *Waiting for Labor to Start* on page 67). During this time progress is slow. Because everyone expects progress after admission to the hospital, it is easy to become discouraged when these hours are spent there, even though little change is normal.

This is a time when labor does not need constant attention. The hours are filled by trying to keep busy, by resting between contractions, and by relaxing—possibly breathing lightly—with them. There is little to entertain you in the hospital, and boredom can drain

> **Labor Stage 1:** The cervix finishes effacing (flattening), and dilates (opens).
>
> *Early phase:* Warm-up contractions, with little change in the cervix.
>
> *Active phase:* With strong contractions, cervix dilates to 6 or 7 centimeters (3 to 3½ fingers).
>
> *Transition:* Strongest contractions of entire labor; complete effacement and dilation.
>
> **Labor Stage 2:** The baby is born.
>
> **Labor Stage 3:** The afterbirth—placenta, bag of waters, and cord—is expelled.
>
> For more details on the stages of labor, please read pages 14 to 19.

the excited, eager energy characteristic of this early waiting time. At home, familiar surroundings promote confidence. There are ways to keep busy and it is natural to remain physically active. Later, when labor demands full attention, hospital surroundings with professional attention at hand may feel more appropriate.

A positive attitude, the release of tension, and physical activity all get labor off to a good start. Should it turn out to be necessary for you to spend labor's early hours in the hospital, bring reading material, games, puzzles, a small radio, even a portable TV to help pass the time pleasantly. At night, do your best to get some sleep.

Once inside the hospital, you and your partner will be settled in a labor room or birthing room, if the

> **Remember:** The warm-up phase takes an average of 8 or 9 hours with a first baby, and about half as long if the mother has had other babies. Contractions last 30 to 60 seconds and are mild to moderate in strength, with rest periods of 5 minutes or longer between contractions.

hospital has one and you chose to be there. In large hospitals, mothers may be admitted to an admitting room and then taken to the labor or birthing room.

A few hospitals and birthing centers have gardens or special sitting rooms where laboring mothers and their helpers can pass the time. Occasionally a shower or bath is available for the mother, in which she can relax, along with her coach. Usually a small chair or stool is placed in the shower. Coaches can put on scrub clothes—the loose-fitting delivery-room clothes worn by doctors and nurses—while mothers wear anything comfortable, including nothing at all.

If you have chosen a **birthing room**, this will be your headquarters for the entire labor and delivery. Birthing rooms are private. Yours may be small or large in size, simply or grandly furnished, with extra floor space to walk around. Usually there is a couch or comfortable chair. Some hospitals admit mothers to the labor room first, and later to the birthing room. Some permit the birthing room to be used only under certain circumstances. Find out what your hospital's policy is. See the list of questions you might ask on page 287.

Labor rooms, often sparsely furnished, may be shared with one or more other women. Space to move around is usually limited. A curtain pulled around your partner's bed creates a certain amount of privacy.

- Doing your team work in front of people you don't know may feel awkward. Keep in mind that coping with labor is your main concern. Thinking about what you can do for your partner will help your self-consciousness to fade into the background. The more you and your partner concentrate on working together, the less you will feel intruded upon by other people around you.

Walking about encourages active contractions. It increases circulation, and good circulation brings oxygen and nutrients to the hard-working uterus while it carries away waste products. When they are up and walking, many women discover that contractions are more comfortable. For some, lying down seems to bring about the opposite effect. As long as it is comfortable for the mother to do so, walking is highly recommended.

- If it is permitted to stroll around together, go to the nursery to look at the babies. Visit the room where your partner will stay after the baby's birth. Be sure to ask the labor nurse before you leave the labor and delivery area.

- Stop for contractions. Your partner may want to sit down or remain standing, possibly leaning against you. You can brace yourself against a wall for better balance. Keep directing her in 4-point releasing all the time.

If your partner must remain in bed, she still can stimulate circulation by changing positions from time to time, moving her arms and legs frequently, and wiggling her fingers, toes, and feet.

- Encourage your partner to relax physically and be calm so that she can tune into her own body.

Your partner is the best judge of the positions and activities that suit her best. Finding a comfortable position during contractions may be easy at first, then more difficult with stronger contractions. She may prefer to alternate walking, sitting, lying down, squatting, being on her hands and knees, or rocking in a rocking chair.

- You may need to try out different ideas until you find one that works. At times, no position will be completely comfortable. Suggest that your partner choose the one that is least objectionable, and then relax into it.

- For whichever position she chooses, try pillows under her legs (if permitted), under her arms and behind her back for support. Keep joints—elbows, wrists, knees—slightly bent for easier relaxation. Feel confident about offering suggestions based on your own observations.

□ □ □

"We found that we needed more than the two pillows given us by the hospital, so I rolled up my shirt and jacket to improvise a bolster or two."

□ □ □

Playing cards or other games, or reading to your partner are good time passers. On the other hand, your partner may find that these disturb her concentration. She may work best with quiet and little or no activity.

- Talk together about what suits her. What works or doesn't work now may change later, so check with her again from time to time.

You and your partner can **take naps** if contractions are mild or the intervals are long, or if labor stops altogether for a while. You might be able to lie down together. If not, and if the only available furniture is a straight-back chair—and you do not want to leave to rest—try this: Pull the chair up facing the bed, adjust the level of the bed so you can sit in the chair and lean forward comfortably, resting your arms on the mattress and your head on your arms. Short naps can do wonders to supply you both with short energy spurts. The key to getting the most out of your rest periods is 4-point releasing, for you as well as your partner.

The nurse, midwife, or doctor will check the baby's heart, your partner's blood pressure, and the progress of labor with an internal **vaginal or rectal exam** from time to time. (Read Internal Exams on page 206 for details.) To make the exam easier and more accurate, your partner may be asked to assume a semi-reclining position. This may be different from the one she has been using, and less comfortable for her. Especially during active labor moving may seem like an impossible task and your encouragement will be valuable to your partner.

- Between contractions you can assist your partner into the new position. Go slowly. Reassure her that she *can* do it. Remind her that she can be comfortable again very shortly. During the exam, help her with 4-point releasing, concentrating especially on bottom and thighs.

- Guide her in using a breathing skill of her choice, if she finds this useful.

"The nurse always asked me to leave when the doctor was about to make an exam. This was the hardest time for her to keep control with no one to guide her and the distraction of the exam. Finally I asked the doctor if he minded me staying. He had no objection. From my experience, I'd advise any coach to speak up at the beginning."

"I found examinations by the doctor to be a good time to tune up for delivery by watching and asking questions about blood and anything else that concerned me."

□ □ □

> **During any procedure that is especially uncomfortable, talk to your partner calmly, soothingly, and quietly.** Remind her to go with what she is feeling, rather than fighting it.

ACTIVE LABOR (MIDDLE OF STAGE 1)

> **The active phase** typically takes 3 to 6 hours with a first baby, and 1 or 2 hours with later babies. Contractions last 45 to 60 seconds and are moderate or strong, with rest periods of 5 minutes or less between contractions. For details on the physical changes during active labor, see page 14.

As contractions grow stronger, your partner will become more serious, less interested in conversation, more centered on herself. Both of you may be getting tired. Rest between contractions is very important now, to conserve energy for the work to come.

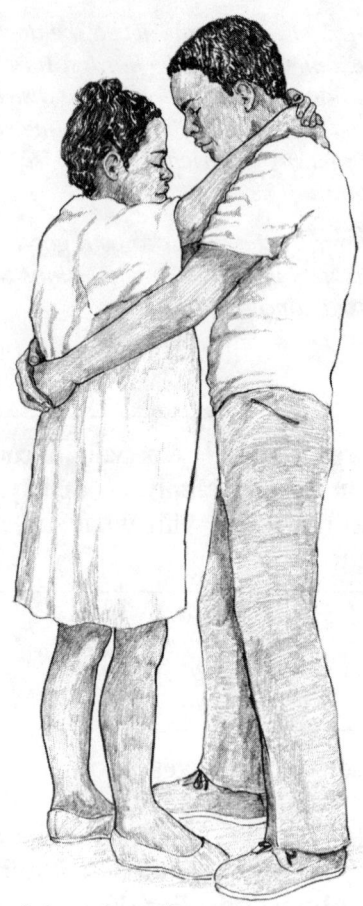

Positions for labor: Standing up

Your partner may be less aware of needing to empty her bladder, as she thinks about how contractions feel.

- Every hour or so, remind her to do this. A full bladder can slow up labor.

- Depending on what her midwife or doctor allows, she may be able to use the bathroom, or she may be required to use the bedpan. In either case, talk with her during a break to prepare her for this move.

- After the next contraction, make your way to the bathroom. Take your time. If she has a contraction on the way she can lean against you while she works with it.

- She may be glad to have you or the nurse stay with her in the bathroom for continuing support. Incidentally, some mothers find sitting on the toilet during labor surprisingly comfortable.

If fluids are allowed, **encourage your partner to sip clear liquids between contractions.** Keeping her fluid level up is important for proper body function.

Finding a position that feels good is worth trying, though it may be impossible to be 100 percent comfortable when contractions are strong. Unless there is a medical reason why the midwife or doctor vetoes a certain position, your partner can try:

1. **Standing up** leaning against you, and sitting down—or remaining standing—during contractions.

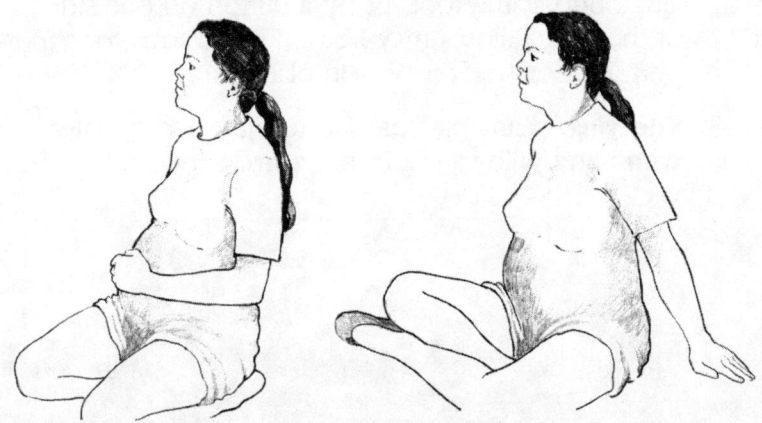

Positions for labor: Kneeling; Indian-style sitting

*Positions for labor:
Semi-reclining*

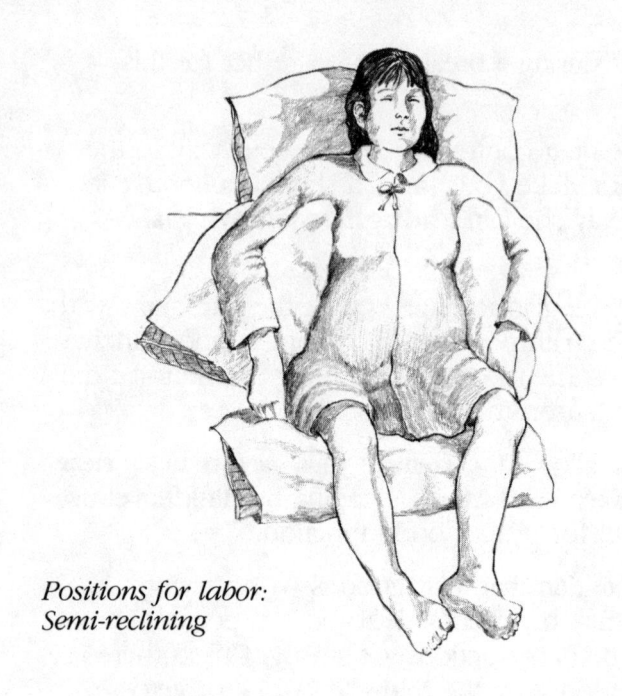

2. **Sitting straight up** or **semi-reclining** with her back supported. The upper half of a hospital bed raises up to form a back rest. It is raised by a crank usually found at the foot, or by a button on one side of the bed. Pillows may be under her arms for support, especially if an IV is in place.

3. **Side lying**, changing from left to right occasionally with extra pillows under her arms, between her

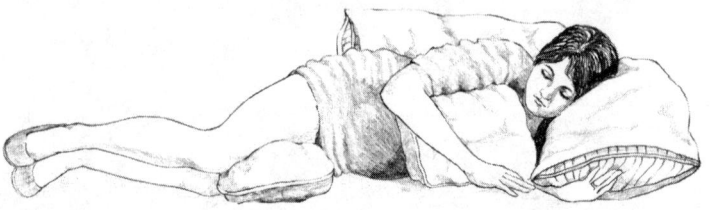

Positions for labor: Side lying

knees, and behind her back, and elbows flexed. When a baby is lying against a mother's back, causing back pain, this position encourages the baby to shift forward against the abdominal wall. See Back Labor, page 244.

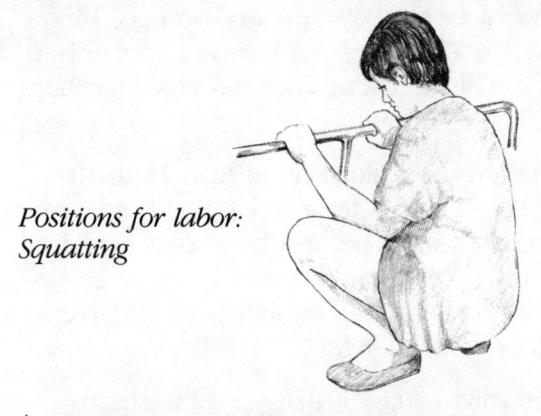

Positions for labor: Squatting

4. **Squatting** on the bed, or on a clean sheet on the floor. The floor is a steadier surface where your partner can feel more securely balanced. In this position she may welcome support for her back from the raised back of her bed, or from you sitting, kneeling, or standing behind her.

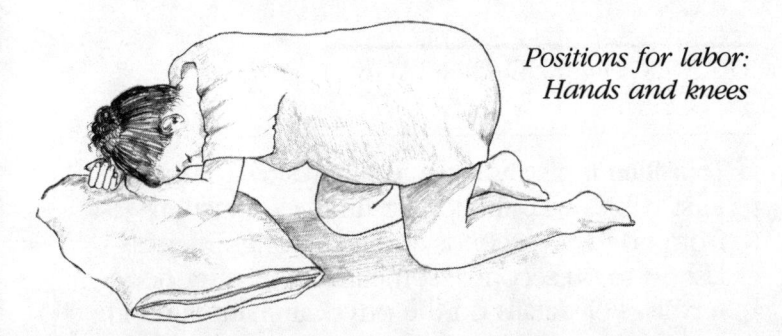

Positions for labor: Hands and knees

5. **On hands and knees**, a position that also can help with backache. If your partner is in a hospital bed,

put up the side rails to help her to feel more secure in this position. It will also lessen the concern of the staff that she might fall out of bed.

Lying flat on her back during labor can lower a mother's blood pressure and slow the flow of blood to her baby, because the weight of the baby presses on large blood vessels in her back. This does not always happen, but it is a possibility. This problem does not arise in other positions.

Suggest that she **try one position for at least 15 to 20 minutes** before she switches to another. She has to get used to it and relax with it before she knows for sure that it won't work. Of course, there is a difference between a position that is questionably uncomfortable and one that is obviously awful.

- Later on, you might suggest that your partner try the discarded position again. Needs change as labor progresses.

> **Remember** that varying positions from time to time also keeps up good circulation.

TRANSITION (END OF STAGE 1)

> **Transition** typically takes 5 minutes to 2 hours. First babies take the longer time. Contractions last from 60 to 90 seconds and are strong. Intervals last 30 to 60 seconds; sometimes there are no intervals. For details on the physical changes during transition, see page 15.

Transition is likely to be your busiest time. Long, difficult contractions punctuated by the briefest of rest periods demand a lot of your partner. The balancing act—staying in control versus giving in to pain—requires continuous effort from you both.

For you, it may be difficult to witness your partner in pain and frustrating that you cannot lessen it somehow. You may be tired and discouraged. Yet this is when she needs help the most.

The nurse, midwife, or doctor may predict how much time transition will take. Though their predictions are based on experience, they are still guesses. You can work most effectively with transition—and so can your partner—if you take one contraction at a time. Even if you could know exactly how long it will last, looking ahead wastes energy. It only makes you wish time would go by faster. It is more effective to focus on the present moment and cope directly with what is happening at each instant. Please read about *Coping with Pain* on page 187, and do not hesitate to ask for assistance from the staff if you need it. It does not diminish your importance, but shows your good sense in making use of all possible resources for your partner's sake.

The arrival of transition is sometimes a surprise. Contractions may suddenly become stronger and longer, instead of building up steadily over a period of time. Out of the blue you might be criticized for something you have been doing all along that, until now, has been well received. Your touch suddenly may be too heavy or too light. Your partner may tell you that you are talking too much, or too loudly. She may feel cold and ask for extra blankets. A few minutes later she may feel too warm and want them removed. She may ask for things and then act surprised or annoyed when she gets them. Remember, it is the demands of labor that produce these reactions, not you.

Transition has many identifying signs. Your partner probably will experience some of them, possibly all of them. Occasionally, labor continues unchanged until a sudden urge to push announces that full dilation has been reached without warning.

□ □ □

"I went from hot to cold and was extremely disoriented, also very bitchy, yelling at Martin to stay away from me."

"I try sucking on a lemon for my thirst and promptly throw up and begin shaking all over. We must be in transition!"

"I gave in to the trembling and relaxed considerably."

□ □ □

SIGNS OF TRANSITION

Burping and hiccoughing are common. Usually they are not uncomfortable and will stop on their own. Accept them and continue working.

Your partner's **vaginal discharge** (mucus-y bleeding from the stretching cervix), with amniotic fluid if the water bag has broken, will increase. If you offer to change the absorbent pads under her, she may feel that raising her hips is impossible and she hasn't an ounce of energy to spare.

- You and the nurse working together can make this task quick and easy.

She may feel **nauseated**, and throw up. If this happens during a contraction it makes control very difficult.

- Encourage her to remain as relaxed as possible and to breathe when she can. Sitting straight up with back support might be the most workable position.

- Encourage her to let whatever is happening, happen, because it becomes harder to handle if she fights it.

- She may feel better if she rinses her mouth with water or mouthwash, or if her face is wiped with a cold, wet cloth. Basins usually are found inside bedside stands, or call the nurse and ask for one.

She may get **the shakes**, especially in her legs. This usually happens between contractions.

- Gently rest your hands on her thighs or stroke them with a gentle, firm motion down toward her feet.

- Remind her to let go of tension, especially in her bottom and thighs. This may ease, though not stop, the shaking.

Fatigue may make your partner feel that responding to another contraction is impossible.

- No matter how short the intervals, insist that she use them to rest.

- Let the cleansing breath that ends a contraction signal the immediate start of 4-point releasing.

- A cold, wet washcloth on her forehead during intervals can be enormously refreshing.

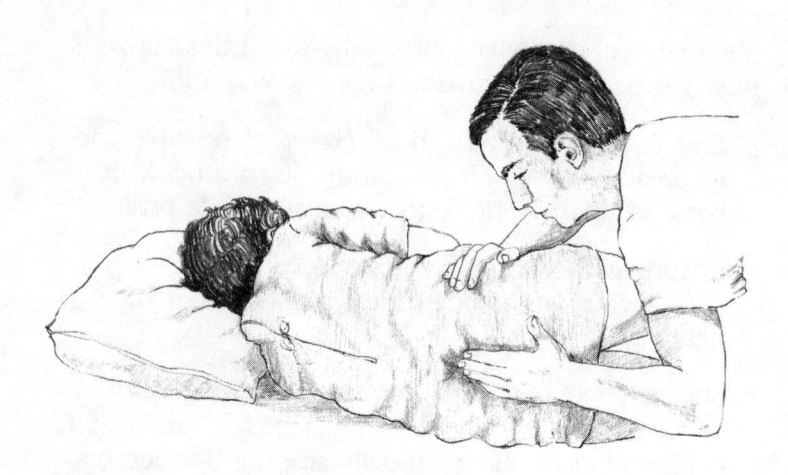

Back pressure may help during Transition

Backache often sets in as the baby moves down, putting temporary pressure on the mother's spine.

- A new position, back pressure, and/or hot or cold compresses may help your partner to carry on through back pain. (Also read Back Labor on page 244.)

☐ ☐ ☐

"I felt very left out and powerless. I was beginning to be exhausted. Every time I would sit down or step into the hall Cathy would yell 'PUSH' and I would jump on the bed and apply HEAVY pressure to her lower back while breathing with her. This stage was not very rewarding for me."

☐ ☐ ☐

With **medication**, your partner may fall asleep directly after each contraction. Usually the next contraction will waken her and she will slip automatically into her breathing. If she has difficulty waking up:

- When contractions come in a regular pattern, you can predict the starting time of each. Alert her 10 seconds before the next contraction is due to start. Touch her shoulder. Call her by name. Speak firmly. Suggest that she take a cleansing breath in preparation. Then, when the contraction comes on, she is already focused and working.

- If your partner is very sleepy, it may help to smooth a wet, cold washcloth over her face, while speaking her name and telling her that you are using the wet cloth to help her awaken.

- If the pattern is irregular, ask your nurse, midwife, or doctor to tell you when a contraction starts by feeling your partner's abdomen. You may be able to do this yourself. Touch must be sensitive and gentle.

□ □ □

"She would awaken at the height of a contraction and frequently fall asleep before she took her cleansing breath. I was very much afraid that she wouldn't be alert during Stage 2 and I felt guilty at allowing her to miss the birth. But as soon as Cynthia started to push, her own body overpowered the Demerol."

□ □ □

Your partner may become very discouraged, certain that she cannot make it to the end, angry about the continuing pain, and frightened that she is being overwhelmed. Many women express these feelings indirectly by being supercritical and irritable.

- Women who are trained to work with their contractions do not expect themselves to make noise, but sometimes yelling or crying a bit can relieve tension.

- If your partner does this, or acts in any other way that you don't expect, you may wonder whether she is helping or hindering herself. During a break, ask her which is happening, and whether she needs your help.

When contractions are strong and difficult to handle, your guidance must be even stronger. Your partner may find it very helpful if you breathe with her. It is easier for her to stay in control by following your example than by struggling alone.

- Get her attention by speaking her name. It may help to touch her shoulder or hand.

- Have her look directly at you and copy you. Continue the breathing she has been using. Try to match her pace. At the same time, remember the important rule of thumb:

  Deep breathing must be **slow** breathing
  Rapid breathing must be **shallow** breathing

- Be firm. You may need to raise your voice and speak commandingly. At all times speak lovingly.

- For a review of breathing techniques and coaching, see page 29.

□ □ □

"Molly used a finger-snapping in tempo to get me breathing. When I broke, I'd have a spell of exasperation and almost quit, then I'd come back with real strong emergency breathing."

"Only a few times did I start to lose control. Then my husband would do the breathing right in my face. It was so annoying

that I would go back to the breathing just to make him stop blowing in my face."

"I really had to work to keep my wife from losing control. If I held her face firmly in one hand and forced her to look at my forehead we could just make it through a contraction."

☐ ☐ ☐

Should your partner feel the urge to push, help her to do her no-push breathing until she receives permission to push. Most likely this will be after she is given a vaginal exam to learn whether she is fully dilated. The urge can be overwhelming and she may have difficulty resisting it.

- Call the nurse, midwife, or doctor and ask for the exam.
- Breathe with her. Ask her to look at you and copy you.

☐ ☐ ☐

"At one point the doctor examined Anna and said, 'You can push when you feel the urge.'"

☐ ☐ ☐

BIRTH (STAGE 2)

> **Stage 2, birth**, typically takes 5 minutes to 2 hours. First babies take longer than later babies do. Contractions last 45 to 60 seconds and are moderate to strong, with rest periods of 2 to 4 minutes between contractions.

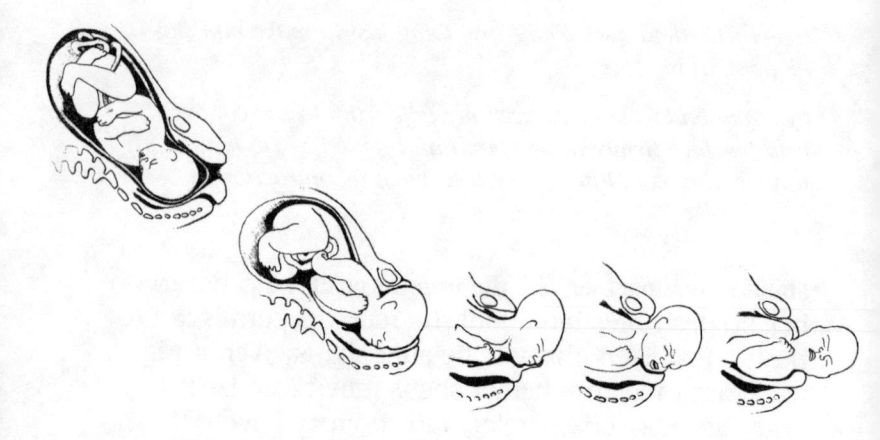

Progress of labor during Stage 2, birth. The baby moves

After transition, the cervix has dilated fully. The baby moves out of the uterus, down through the vagina, and is born. The vagina, and the perineum too, are made of wonderful elastic tissue that stretches with every push. Usually this process is slow but sure, although it may move along quickly. Pushing for the birth itself takes only a few minutes. Your guidance and praise, and that of the staff, will help your partner to push effectively.

During the interval before the first pushing contraction, quickly and simply review the pushing position and how to push with your partner. For additional details on pushing and coaching to help pushing, review the *Quick Guide to Pushing* on page 164, and *Mother's Skills,* pages 21 to 66.

Some women hold back against opening up to let the baby out. Your partner may tighten up instead of letting go—and no wonder! She may find it hard to abandon her modesty, with her legs apart. The skin of the stretching perineum burns and feels as though it

down through the open cervix, turns slightly, and is born.

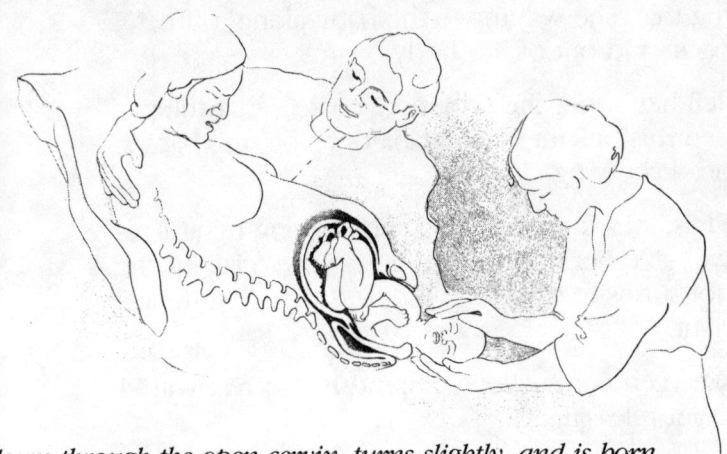

will split. Her lower back may feel as though it will break. The pressure of the baby's head inside may feel like an enormous bowel movement about to come out. The urge to push is a tremendous force and it can be scary to feel it taking over.

She needs encouragement to work with her body instead of against it. To help, you must consider her feelings. The nurse, midwife, or doctor can offer suggestions, too.

- If she has a bowel movement (which sometimes happens), the nurse will clean it away. Tell her no one minds. The important thing is to get the baby out.

- Tell her the pressure she feels is the stretching of her perineum, giving the baby room to get out. Though she hurts, her body is not being harmed.

- Remind her to push through her pain, not to be afraid of it, to open up to it and go with it. By doing that, she will move the baby along, off her back, and out of her body.

- Tell her about the progress you see, that the perineum is bulging, the vagina opening, the baby's head showing.

- Praise her for everything she is doing right. This will give her the heart to go on, especially if she is not sure she is making progress or doing things right.

- Between contractions, remind her to rest with 4-point releasing.

If your partner's pushes are too short to move the baby along, you will know because the staff will tell her.

- Have her push as you count slowly up to 5 or 10. Of course, she can push longer if it feels right to do it.

- If you want to tell her to continue the push, as she pushes avoid saying "hold it" because this often translates into holding back with the muscles of the perineum. Instead, try "keep going" or "continue."

□ □ □

"I spent over an hour in the shower with the hot water hitting my back—I alternated between pushing in a crouched position and resting in a seated position. This was a tremendous help."

"At the nurse's suggestion, I found it was easiest to push as I held her hands. She (and later Sam) would pull back very hard toward herself as I would pull hard in my direction."

"This nurse and a student had me put my feet on their waists to push."

"During each contraction, I would lift her back and have her push her feet against my other arm. We were finally moving."

"Pushing was a relief. Suddenly Madeline didn't need so much coaching. Our baby was about to be born and that was fantastic. I wasn't tired any more."

□ □ □

When birth is near, a little bit of the baby will start to show at the outer opening of the vagina. When the opening has widened to the size of a 50-cent piece (this is called *caput*), it is the signal to go to the delivery room, unless your partner is going to give birth in a birthing room. Women who are not first-time mothers may change rooms sooner because their babies usually are born more quickly.

□ □ □

"The baby's head began to show and a little piece of hair stuck out, a tiny curl. I never felt so high in my life."

□ □ □

If your partner is to give birth in her bed, she will remain where she is. Preparations will go on around you both, while you continue to work together. Otherwise, it will be time to move.

If you may wear street clothes in the labor room but must **change for the delivery room**, do it early to avoid last-minute scurry and absence from your partner during this most exciting time.

- Put on your delivery room clothes during labor, by the time your partner has dilated to 5 centimeters, or before transition starts (when you are needed to help and would not want to be away).

- Because you will be holding the baby soon, make sure your hands are washed. Usually, there are sinks in the labor room; there are always sinks directly outside the delivery room. Water for the delivery room sink is turned on by a pedal or knee lever under the sink. Liquid soap may be obtained by pushing a lever, too, although you will probably see individually wrapped packages of small, square brushes on a shelf or dispenser above the sink. Wet a brush and it becomes soapy.

□ □ □

"The nurses prevented Cal from coming into the delivery room because he wasn't wearing sterile garb. (Neither were the doctors—except gloves—or nurses, including the one who held out the baby.) There's no repeating her birth so I guess I will always feel disappointed that Cal missed out because of rules. I felt they could have given him the gown faster and not stalled him so much."

□ □ □

MOVING TO THE DELIVERY ROOM

If she feels like it, your partner may be invited to walk to the delivery room, especially if she is to use a birthing chair. Or she may be transferred in her bed, or asked to move onto a stretcher.

Moving from bed to stretcher to delivery table can be awkward and uncomfortable for a woman about to give birth.

- You can work with the nurses by helping your partner to slide her head and shoulders over first, then her body, and last her legs. During the transfers, the stretcher is held against the bed and later the table.

- Bring along pillows, especially if the delivery table does not have a raised back.
- If your partner wears glasses but does not have them on, bring them with you. It can be upsetting to be cut off from one's surroundings by being unable to see. And your partner should be able to see the baby when she wants to, most likely during birth or immediately afterward.
- Take a wet washcloth to refresh her face and moisten her lips between contractions.
- Don't forget your camera.

For the delivery you may be given a mask, cap, and possibly shoes, all made of cloth or paper. Put on your cap first, then your mask. Then, when you tie the mask strings around your head, they will not tangle in your hair. The metal strip along the top edge of some masks bends to fit over your nose. It keeps the mask in place so it will not slide up into your eyes. If you wear glasses, it prevents them from steaming up every time you exhale. The shoes slip on over your own shoes.

If you and your partner had requested dim lighting and quiet for the birth (see Leboyer, page 219), this is the time to remind the midwife, doctor, or nurse.

Of course, contractions are continuing throughout this busy time.

Your partner may be encouraged to continue pushing or asked to do no-push breathing, depending on how close the baby is to being born. While she still needs support and encouragement, everyone—including you—is likely to be temporarily preoccupied with individual tasks.

- To avoid conflict, try to find out in advance the routine your hospital follows when preparing for a birth and, most important, what is required of you now. Knowing the facts will lessen confusion, and allow you to plan ahead so you can remain by your partner's side while everyone else is busy.

THE DELIVERY

In the birthing or delivery room, coaches usually are asked to stay at the head of the bed or delivery table, or alongside the birthing chair. There is usually a stool for you to sit on. If an anesthetist is present, he will sit near you. Here you are closest to your partner and can encourage her as she works. You can share the birth together.

If she is lying flat and wants to be lifted forward as she pushes or so that she can see the birth, you are in the perfect position to help.

- Between contractions, slide the pillows under your partner's head and shoulders. Ask whether she is comfortable, when she pushes with her next contraction.

POSITIONS

A delivery table, used in a delivery room, is designed so that a woman giving birth lies **on her back**, flat or raised forward at an angle.

A birthing chair, used in the delivery room or in a

birthing room, supports the mother in a **sitting** position and can tilt so that she sits straight up or at any angle.

In a birthing room, one of several positions may be used. The position for pushing the baby to the vaginal opening may differ from the position for birth. Your partner may **sit in bed** with her back raised and her legs relaxed apart on the mattress or up in stirrups. This is the most common position.

She might lie **on her side**.

She might prop herself on her hands and knees. If she is well supported by pillows and a firm mattress, she can relax and not strain to hold herself in position.

Squatting or sitting on a small birthing stool works best on the floor, because mattresses are not steady enough. In this case, clean sheets are spread beneath the mother.

Coaches sometimes support their partners by sitting behind them on the bed or on the floor. The variety of your choices depends on on how familiar and at ease your midwife or doctor is with the positions. Please also read Points about Positions in Chapter 3, page 58.

PREPARATIONS

Depending on the way your hospital does things, preparations for the birth may include a few simple arrangements, or a lot of bustling about. While the midwife or doctor scrubs, a nurse washes your partner's perineum. Your partner's legs are covered with long, loose stockings and placed in stirrups.

The stirrups may be moved wider apart or closer together, forward or back, lower or higher. They must be of equal height to ensure proper circulation as well as comfort.

Straps, sometimes buckled over the legs, must not be uncomfortably tight or they can cause poor circulation and leg cramps.

- If straps are used, ask your partner how they feel. Even though you see that nurses are busy, ask one to loosen too-tight straps.

When a woman is put to sleep for birth, **her arms may be confined** loosely at her sides to keep them from slipping off the table and being injured. There is no reason to confine the arms of a woman who is awake.

If your partner says she has a **leg cramp**, she should straighten her leg and push her heel away from her body while pulling her toes toward her at the same time. Straps must be unbuckled to do this. The nurse may massage the tightened muscle and lower the stirrup for better circulation.

In a delivery room, when a woman gives birth without stirrups, her feet simply remain on the table with her legs apart and her knees bent.

The delivery table is "broken," which means that the lower half is rolled under the upper half by turning a handle at the head of the table.

- You may be asked to turn the handle that breaks the table.

If you are using a **birthing chair,** the midwife or doctor may raise it and tip it back at a slight angle so that she or he can see more easily as the baby is born.

The midwife or doctor will put on sterile gloves and maybe a mask, cap, and sterile gown. If **sterile sheets** are used, this is when they are draped over your partner from the waist down.

- Though your partner may touch the sterile sheets from underneath, remind her not to reach over and touch them from above. This is the "sterile field" and the idea is to keep it as germ free as possible. Suggest that she keep hold of the hand grips or stirrup bars located alongside the delivery table, or attached to the birthing chair seat. You may touch your partner, but remember that you, too, must not touch the sheets.

While all this is going on, **your partner will be pushing** with each contraction, bringing the baby closer to birth.

- Continue your help and encouragement, as you have been doing all along.

She may be greatly heartened if she can watch in a **mirror** and see her baby appear as she opens. Her abdomen is too large for her to look directly down at herself. The mirrors attached to the wall or over the delivery table—the only way a mother can see herself give birth—often need adjusting.

- Ask your partner if she wants to look, and whether she can see. If you put your face next to hers, you can look in the mirror too, and see what she sees.

- Have the nurse tilt the mirror until your partner can see her perineum, or ask if you may do it yourself.

- If you know in advance that there is no mirror, bring a small one from home. A hand mirror is easiest to hold. You or a nurse may be able to hold it so your partner can see her progress.

The professionals with you now may offer encouragement and suggestions to your partner. Along with your guidance, this can give her the cheering-on that she needs.

□ □ □

"I heard some 'good, good' from the background but nothing from the foot of the table. I asked Mrs. Wilson to tell the doctor I needed encouragement. In her straight way she relayed the message (which I had said with some sarcasm), and he started to talk to me."

□ □ □

With each contraction, if you are watching the perineum, you will see more of the baby's head and a steady thinning of the perineum. The midwife or doctor may massage this tissue or place hot compresses against it to help it soften and stretch. From time to time a nurse will listen to the baby's heart.

If an **episiotomy** is made, the perineum is first injected with a medication to numb it. You may be surprised by the large size of the syringe and needle. Remember that the perineum is already greatly numbed by the pressure of the baby against it. Occasionally a mother may feel the episiotomy as it is made, but it takes only a few seconds and is quickly over.

This is the time about which coaches may worry, wondering whether they will feel unwell or nervous. Most find that they are too busy to have time to feel nervous, dizzy, weak, or nauseated. On the chance that this does happen to you, admit it, and get some help.

- If you don't feel well, tell the medical attendant closest to you. Someone will help you to sit down, if you are not sitting already, will lower your head, and bring you smelling salts, a basin, a cold cloth—whatever you need.

You may prefer to leave the room. Usually you are permitted to return when you feel better.

- Take very slow, long, deep breaths and go loose from head to toe. Continue to do this for awhile even after you feel better. Someone will help your partner while you care for yourself. Should you feel embarrassed, remember that many nurses, midwives, and doctors have had the same experience sometime in their careers. Everyone will understand and admire your courage for speaking up.

□ □ □

"I was nervous about the delivery room and I thought I might not be able to hack it. But that was just a flashing thought and we got onto the table and down to business."

"When I saw the baby I felt lightheaded and I said aloud to no one in particular, 'I'm going to pass out.' Two nurses put my head down between my legs and put some smelling salts under my nose and in a few minutes I felt fine. The rest of the time there were no more problems."

□ □ □

As the baby is born, the doctor or midwife will ask your partner not to push. She may be so wrapped up in her work that she doesn't hear the request. It is not easy to make the switch from pushing to no-push breathing. She may need you to guide her.

- Your midwife or doctor may announce during a break that the baby is likely to be born with the next contraction. Before the contraction starts, briefly review the no-push breathing with your partner. Have her look at you while you show her, and perhaps do it together.

- Listen carefully, and as soon as you hear the request to stop pushing, tell your partner to do her no-push breathing. If you breathe with her, she can simply copy you.

◻ ◻ ◻

"She shouts. This time the doctor repeats his instructions to her. I also repeat. The assisting nurse repeats. All is said and we rest for a moment. Our faith is beginning to waver. Maybe we cannot do this. The fourth push is successful. She pushes so hard and so long she gets red-faced—and I see the child. The doctor says 'do not push.' She complies instantly, successfully. Then one final push and it is out. The child is our first son. He cries out. We cry joyous tears, too."

◻ ◻ ◻

At last the baby will ease out. If you are watching, you will see the baby's head turn to one side as it is born. Next comes a shoulder. The rest slides out quickly and easily, in less time than it takes you to read about it.

◻ ◻ ◻

"At the end, Pete was holding me up and yelling 'push harder' and the doctor at the other end was yelling the same thing. We all three were a team, and out popped Andrea. She came out in one fell swoop and the doctor sort of caught her on the fly."

"Frank was watching the delivery through a window. Originally he wanted no part of any of this, but there he was, watching in great excitement."

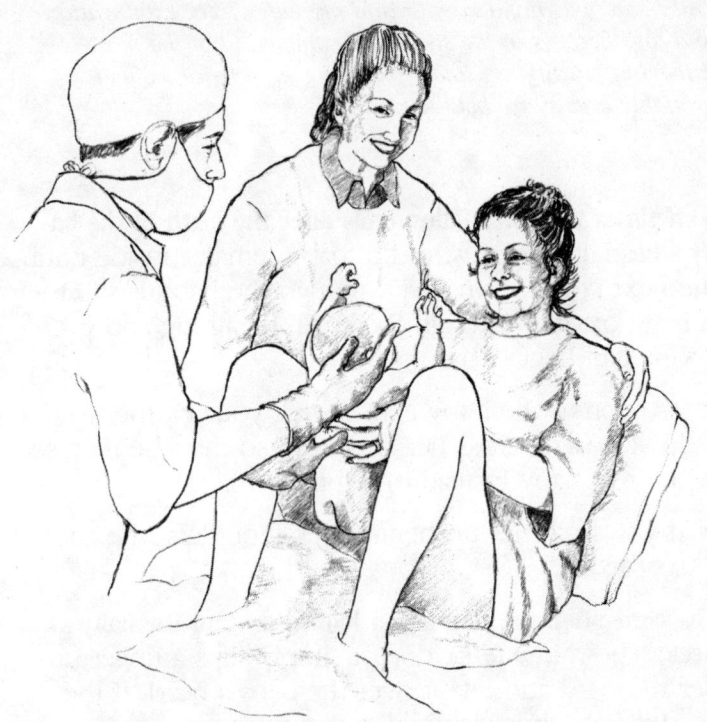

Mothers may reach spontaneously for the baby

"He came out grabbing the cord. The doctor had to unwrap his fingers. He cried right away."

"She had been in distress because the cord had been tightly wrapped around her neck. It didn't seem to affect her any, because she cried right away and turned a beautiful red."

"When he was finally delivered, I was laughing. I was ecstatic for 4 days."

"John didn't realize until after the baby was born that he had been crying."

"All I saw was my daughter and my wife. Total exhilaration and togetherness in the successful completion of the most satisfying, gratifying, and frustrating experience we will probably ever share between us."

□ □ □

Sometimes the contraction ends after the birth of the baby's head and the rest of the baby remains inside until the next contraction. Even though the baby is still receiving oxygen through the cord, breathing and even crying can begin now.

- As soon as the baby is born, tell your partner to look down across her abdomen so that she may see the real baby instead of a mirror image.

- If you hold her up behind her shoulders, she can see better.

The cord often may be found looped around the baby's neck. The midwife or doctor simply slips a finger under the cord and lifts it over the baby's head. If the cord is tight, it is clamped and cut instead.

In this thrilling moment your partner may reach out spontaneously for the baby.

- When sterile sheets are used, you will have to remind her to keep her hands under the sheets until the baby is laid above the sheets on her chest. This restriction is easier to remember if she holds onto the hand grips.

The birth of a baby is a very moving experience, even for the medical attendants who have seen it many times. You may be so deeply touched that you find yourself in tears. Don't let the lack of privacy keep you from hugging and kissing your partner if this is what seems natural to do.

□ □ □

"I cried like a baby when our child was born. In talking with other men, I find this is a common reaction. It felt great to release all the emotions that had built up for so long—9 months."

□ □ □

Quick Coaching Guide (Early and Active Labor)

For all labor:

- 4-point releasing is the foundation.
- Breathings are slow and deep, or rapid and shallow.
- Work with, not against, contractions.
- Physical activity balanced with rest promotes progress.
- In early labor, nourishment (if allowed) supplies energy. In active labor, give clear liquids in sips or ice chips between contractions (if allowed).
- Prevent boredom, which drains energy, promotes anxiety. At home, keep mildly busy. In the hospital use games, reading, to pass the time.

Positions:

- Changes from time to time promote labor.
- Use pillows, back support for comfort.
- Try one position for 15 to 20 minutes before changing, unless it is obviously uncomfortable. If it doesn't work the first time, try the position again later.

Hospital procedures:

- Request that procedures be delayed until a contraction is over (a possible exception is a vaginal exam).
- Encourage 4-point releasing during procedures.
- Encourage breathing skills if necessary.

Quick Coaching Guide (Transition)

During transition:

- Accept what happens, and deal with one thing at a time.

    Backache: Have your partner choose a position that will ease pressure on her back (side lying, hands-and-knees, sitting, or standing and leaning forward). With your hands, apply strong, steady pressure against the parts of her back that hurt.

    Burping and hiccoughing: Relax and accept it.

    Fatigue: Complete rest between contractions; encouragement and 4-point releasing during contractions.

    Chills; feeling too warm: Ask for extra blankets; ask for cold water to sponge your partner's face, neck, arms. Remember that changing from cold to hot and back again is common and normal.

    Discouragement, irritability: Work contraction by contraction, rest period by rest period. Remind your partner that you are getting closer to your goal, the baby's birth.

Nausea and vomiting: Help your partner to relax as much as possible. Have her rinse her mouth. Wipe her face with a wet cloth.

Shaking: 4-point releasing. Use your hands to stroke or support shaking legs.

Urge to push: Coach your partner in no-push breathing until she receives permission to push. Ask for a vaginal exam to see if the cervix has reached 10 centimeters, or 5 fingers dilation.

For yourself:

- Keep your ego out of coaching.
- Take breaks when you need them. Ask the nurse to coach during your absence.
- Use 4-point releasing.
- Remember what you are working for, the baby's birth.

Quick Coaching Guide (Pushing)

You can help during pushing with:

- **Encouragement, information, and praise.**
  "You can do it."
  "Let yourself go with the pushing urge."
  "Don't be afraid, push *through* the pain."

"Take each contraction as it comes."
"I can see *this much* [making a circle with thumb and forefinger] of the baby's head."
"You are wonderful."
"What a hard worker you are! Bravo!"

- **Physical support.**

    Basics: Support parts of her body (back and legs especially) when they are not otherwise supported, to save her from fatigue.

- **Directions.**

    Basics: Remind her to tilt her head forward and round her shoulders and arms to help round her back.
    Remind her to let her mouth fall open slightly to help her relax her bottom.
    Remind her to feel her abdominal muscles tighten as she pushes, helping to give power to her pushes.
    Remind her to tilt her head back for air exchanges.
    Remind her to make each push long enough to get the baby moving.
    Remind her to concentrate the power of her push down, through, and out her bottom, aiming for a target if this helps.
    Remind her to open up her bottom.
    Remind her to rest completely between contractions.

- **Comfort.**

    Basics: A wet washcloth to refresh her face and neck between contractions; Vaseline or Chapstick for dry lips; ice chips or sips of water or tea with honey for dry mouth (if permitted).

Quick Coaching Guide (Birth)

Locations:
Labor or birthing bed, delivery table, birthing chair.

Positions:
Semi-reclining, side-lying, hands and knees, squatting with or without a birthing stool.

Reminders:

- Wash your hands now so that you can hold the baby after birth.
- Bring your partner's eyeglasses, pillows, wet washcloth to the delivery room.
- Remind midwife or doctor of dim lighting if you have requested it.
- Check your partner's comfort, particularly with stirrup adjustments and leg straps.
- If there is a mirror, ask that it be adjusted so that your partner can see the birth.

Directions:

- Continue pushing reminders.
- Support your partner physically if she needs it.
- Review and be prepared to use no-push breathing for the birth.

- Be prepared to remind your partner and yourself to avoid touching sterile sheets.

If you feel dizzy or faint:

- Don't be embarrassed; take care of yourself.
- Take very slow, long, deep breaths.
- Sit down and put your head between your knees.
- Tell a member of the staff how you are feeling, especially if you want further help for yourself or for your partner.

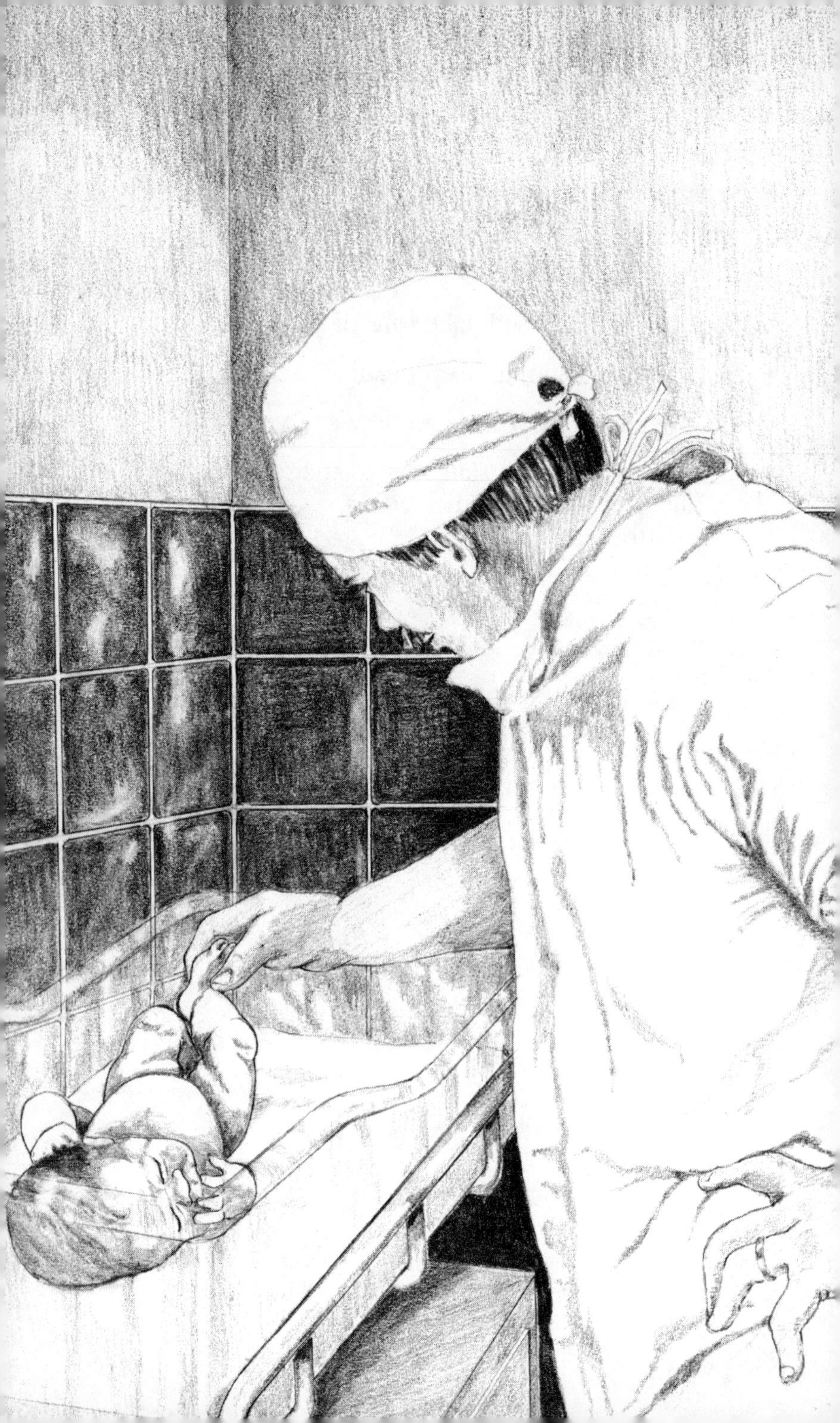

8. The Coach's Skills (After the Birth)

Newborn babies look surprisingly different from the pink, plump babies in advertisements, or from the babies of your friends. They may be limp with slightly grey or blue coloring until breathing begins, when they are transformed by varying shades of rose. Babies of parents with dark skin may be pale in color for the first few hours or days of life. These babies often have dark blue to purple spots (Mongolian spots) over their backs and buttocks. This concentrated pigment usually disappears or merges with the final skin coloring within 1 to 5 years. They undergo the same kinds of changes in coloring at birth. Hands and feet may remain dusky for a short while. Sometimes patches of vernix, nature's skin cream for babies, cover the skin along with streaks of blood from the mother's cervix.

□ □ □

"His skin was smooth, pink, and wet, and as clean as though he had just come out of a bath. The nurse told me I had a beautiful child, and I nodded in total agreement."

"I lifted my head and there she was, all red and messy and gorgeous. I had thought that before she was cleaned up I would be repulsed, but to me she was the most beautiful sight in the world."

"The baby was sitting in the doctor's hand. She came out with her face all screwed up and she was blue-white. The doctor

rubbed her back and the most beautiful moment of all occurred. As she began to cry we actually saw her body turn pink all over from the head to her feet."

"The baby was purple upon delivery, and in respiratory distress. I actually used 4-point releasing to calm myself and not panic about the baby. It worked."

☐ ☐ ☐

The first step in attending to a newborn is to clear the nose and mouth of fluids with a bulb syringe or plastic tube so that breathing will be easier.

Often babies breathe and cry on their own, directly after birth. If the baby is not yet breathing, the midwife or doctor may stimulate breathing by rubbing the baby's back or feet. Spanking babies is more often seen in the movies than in real life.

Next, **the cord is cut**, unless you and your partner have asked to have this step delayed until the pulsing stops. Transfusion of extra blood from the placenta through the cord to the baby—the reason one medical opinion supports the delay—can happen only if the baby is held lower than the mother. A differing medical opinion notes that the transfusion demands extra effort from the baby, to adjust to the extra blood volume.

- If you want to cut the cord yourself, ask the midwife or doctor ahead of time or it is likely to be done before you realize it.

The cord is amazing to see, particularly when you imagine the three blood vessels inside that have given the baby life. It is spiralled and taut while the blood is still circulating, or limp after it has stopped, and about the thickness of your thumb. Its color may be whitish-yellow or bluish-grey.

At this point **the baby may be placed in a nearby crib** that is heated and equipped with light, oxygen, and electric suction. Some doctors put newborns directly in the crib as a matter of routine, and others do it for special reasons only. For example, an otherwise healthy baby who is slow to begin breathing might be taken to the crib and given oxygen.

Otherwise, **the baby is now placed in your partner's arms**. In the absence of sterile sheets, your partner and you may have been touching and holding the baby long before this point. At the time of birth, a woman may reach down and help to lift the baby out of her body.

- You can help your partner to hold the baby, who will be wet and slippery.

Your partner can feel the baby's warmth and movement directly against her own skin, if her gown has been removed. A brand-new baby does not have enough energy to stabilize breathing and circulation, and to keep warm, too. When a baby and mother, both nude, are wrapped together in heated blankets, the mother's body heat creates an excellent incubator.

- Be sure the baby's head is covered to prevent loss of this precious heat. Leave an opening for the face to permit easy breathing. Some birthing centers and hospitals supply tiny hats for newborns.

Juggling your role as coach and photographer can be a challenge. You will not be able to do both at once. You will have to use on-the-spot judgment about when you can be spared to take a picture.

- You might ask a nurse or other medical attendant to

substitute temporarily for you, either as coach or as photographer.

- Ask your partner if she can spare you. She may be able to, especially during delivery when the midwife or doctor often does a lot of coaching.
- Get permission from the midwife or doctor before you walk around the delivery room. To be on the safe side, avoid touching anything unless you have been told specifically that you may.

> **The afterbirth**—placenta, water bag, and the remainder of the cord—typically is passed 5 to 30 minutes after the birth. The one or two contractions last 15 to 30 seconds and are mild to moderate. For details on the mother's physical changes during the third stage, see page 18.

The midwife or doctor may order some **medication for your partner** to help her uterus expel the afterbirth, after the baby's birth, during the last stage of labor. It is given as an injection or through the IV if there is one. For details, please read about medications on page 221.

Breastfeeding has the same effect, because it stimulates the mother's body to produce a hormone that contracts the uterus. Many, but not all, babies are keen to nurse soon after birth. However, many hospital birthing routines do not include putting the baby to the mother's breast immediately after birth, but wait instead until the baby has been examined and the episiotomy has been repaired.

The afterbirth detaches from the inside of the uterus and is passed easily out through the vagina assisted by one or two mild to moderate contractions.

You may be interested to see **the placenta, the bag of water that surrounds it, and the remainder of the cord** that attaches at its center. The placenta is reddish-brown, round—about 10 inches across—and thick, with shiny, uneven surfaces. On one side you can see several blood vessels that channel into the cord, like little roads leading to three main highways.

- If you ask, your midwife or doctor will explain what you are looking at and how this marvelous organ served the baby during pregnancy. You need not feel that you *must* look, just as a mother need not feel she must watch her baby's birth in a mirror. These are your personal choices.

□ □ □

"The afterbirth came out within seconds after the cord was cut."

"The placenta took 35 minutes. All that time the doctor was sewing up the episiotomy."

"The contractions stopped abruptly after birth and the placenta was helped out by an attendant who massaged my stomach despite my loud complaints."

□ □ □

Once the afterbirth is expelled, some doctors examine the inside of the uterus by hand to make sure no fragments of the placenta remain behind. (The placenta itself is examined for the same reason.) Such an examination can be painful.

- You can help your partner by talking her through 4-point releasing—concentrating especially on her bottom and thighs—and a breathing of her choice.

- Remind her that the exam takes only a few seconds. The more she can go with it, opening her body to it, the quicker it will pass.

□ □ □

"I was sort of spaced on the baby, forgetting Sarah for a moment. After the baby was disconnected I realized that she was in pain, so we started emergency breathing."

□ □ □

Next, if one was made, **the episiotomy will be repaired**. This stitching might take around 30 minutes. Your partner may feel the stitching and involuntarily tighten her bottom and lift her buttocks off the table. You might hear the midwife or doctor ask her to relax. She is uncomfortable and tired by now, and this is hard to do. She may have another injection to further numb her perineum.

- Guide her through 4-point releasing.

- If you encourage her to look at the baby, or to talk with you about the labor, she may be able to ignore the stitching.

- Should she get the shakes or feel chilly, both common at this time, ask for more warmed blankets to put around her. Relaxing usually helps, and the warmth of your hand touching her does too.

- If she is too preoccupied, she may want you to hold the baby until the stitching is finished.

After the episiotomy is repaired, your partner may stretch out her legs and make herself comfortable. If she is on a delivery table, it will be restored to its former length with the stirrups removed.

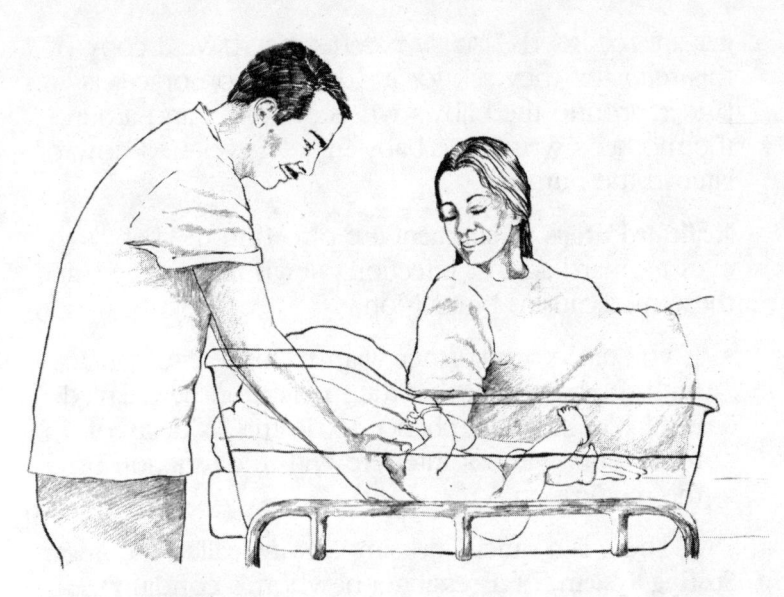

A Leboyer bath

If you and your partner have requested a **Leboyer bath** (read about the Leboyer Method on page 219 for details), it may be done during the episiotomy repair or afterward. Sometimes a heater is brought in along with the bath basin. You, your partner, or both of you together might give the bath. Even if you have held newborns before, you may wonder how to get a safe grip on this slippery little baby.

- Ask the medical attendants for suggestions about giving the bath so that you can feel confident and enjoy the baby's reaction.

The baby will receive an injection of **Vitamin K** shortly after delivery, to help the blood-clotting system to work properly.

Footprints and a print of the mother's right forefinger are recorded. Usually parents may have a copy of this record if they ask for it. Identification bracelets are placed around the baby's wrists or ankles and around the mother's wrist. The baby may be weighed now or later in the nursery.

Medicated drops or ointment are placed in the baby's eyes to guard against infection. Newborns can see, and these medications blur vision.

- If you and your partner want to make eye contact with the baby, ask that the medication be delayed until you have the chance to do this. A delay of up to 2 hours will not interfere with the function of the medication.

There is a quick and simple way, called the **Apgar Scoring System,** of assessing a newborn's condition. One minute after birth, 5 minutes later, and sometimes again in 10 minutes, the baby's color, reflexes, breathing, heart rate, and muscle tone are noted. Each of these 5 characteristics receives 0 to 2 points for each exam. The points are added together to make a score of up to 10 points for each exam. The final 3 score numbers are written as a fraction (for example: 8/9/10), a kind of shorthand message to give information about the newly born baby to the pediatrician and nursery nurses who may not see her until she arrives in the nursery 1 or 2 hours after birth.

A healthy baby can lose a point or two on color or breathing, especially in the first minute or so of life outside the protection of the uterus.

A pediatrician may examine the baby now, or later in the nursery.

- Watch this examination if you can, and ask ques-

APGAR SCORING SYSTEM

Characteristic	0	1	2
Color	Blue, pale	Body, pink extremities pale	Body completely pink
Respiratory Effort	Absent	Slow, irregular, weak cry	Strong cry
Heart Rate	Absent	Less than 100	More than 100
Muscle Tone	Limp	Some flexing of extremities	Active Motion
Reflex Irritability	Absent	Grimace	Cry

Apgar Chart

tions if you feel like it. It is a good opportunity to learn a lot about the baby.

If the baby is a boy and a **circumcision** is planned, the obstetrician may do it now or after 12 to 72 hours, depending on his custom. Traditionally, Jewish babies are circumcised on the 7th day after birth. For details on circumcision, read page 220.

RECOVERY (OBSERVATION) PERIOD

The next hour or two is an observation period. During this time a nurse keeps an eye on your partner's blood pressure and her vaginal flow. A sanitary pad is worn now.

With her hand on your partner's abdomen, **the nurse feels to make sure the uterus is contracted and firm.** This is called "checking the fundus" (as the body of the uterus is named). If the uterus relaxes, which can cause unnecessary bleeding, it will be massaged. The uterus can be very tender after birth, and both the exam and the massage may be painful for your partner.

- Once again, remind her to concentrate on 4-point releasing and, if she needs it, a light easy breathing.

◻ ◻ ◻

"After the baby was born Elaine massaged her for 15 or 20 minutes, then I gave her a bath for a half hour. We all had champagne and all the nurses came in (and a couple of doctors too) and I felt we were all having a great party, together in the recovery room. We all hugged and snuggled for about an hour."

◻ ◻ ◻

Most hospitals encourage mother and baby to remain together, along with the coach, during this observation period, although it may be the policy of some hospitals to take the baby to the nursery now. The nurse who watches over your partner will keep an eye on the baby as well. The three of you may be transferred to a recovery room or you may stay in the delivery or birthing room. If you are in a birthing center, you probably will stay in the room where the baby was born until it is time to go home, within 12 to 24 hours. Family and close friends may be able to join you briefly for a short visit. Remember that this is a time for you and your partner to rest, hold the baby, and enjoy each other.

- Your partner might appreciate a fresh gown and a warm sweater and socks.

- Family and friends can be called if a phone is within reach.

- Mothers often feel hungry and thirsty after giving birth. If permitted, a light snack could taste wonderful for everyone—juice, tea, a light soup, toast, crackers, and champagne! Your place of birth may provide these, or you may want to plan ahead and bring them with you when you first arrive in labor (see page 295 for lists of things you might like to bring with you to the hospital). At that time, the nurse can tell you where to keep them until you are ready for them.

If your partner is planning to nurse the baby, this is the best time to begin.

- Nurses, midwives, and doctors can offer practical suggestions to mothers who are breastfeeding for the first time. Ask for pointers.

- The most comfortable position for early nursing is usually side-lying or semi-reclining, especially when a new episiotomy is sore.

- Not all new babies feel like sucking right away. Remind your partner not to be discouraged or feel rejected if the baby is not interested on this first try.

Holding a baby is a delight, because they are such wonderfully solid, warm little bundles of life. Although newborns look astonishingly tiny, they are surprisingly sturdy. While gentleness is important, they can and should be held firmly. For your first time, sit down and ask the nurse to hand you the baby. Take hold of

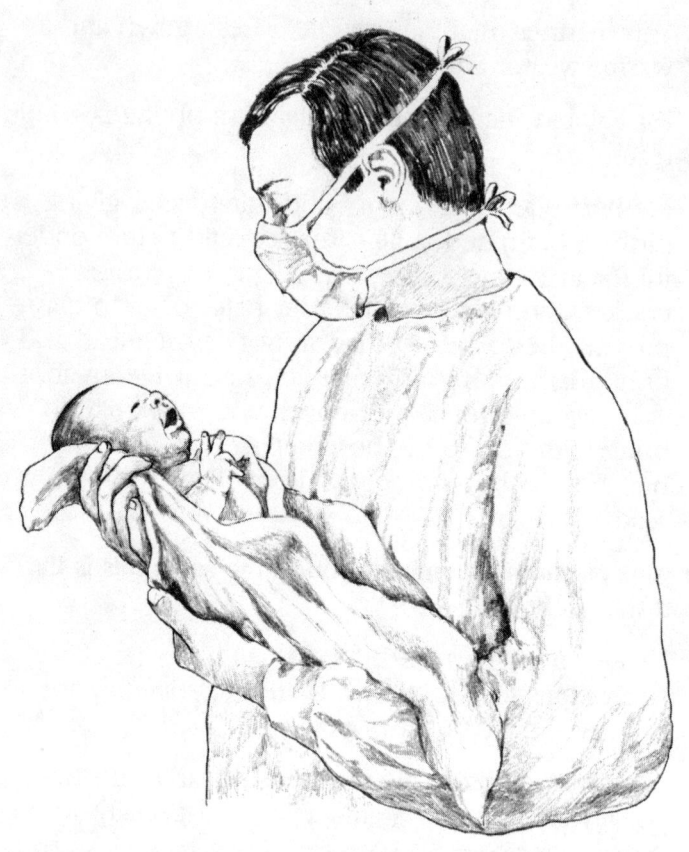

Cradle the baby's head and shoulders in one hand, his lower back and bottom in the other.

this baby with confidence. Cradle the head, neck, and shoulders in one hand and grasp the lower back and buttocks with the other. Relax, look at each other, and enjoy yourselves.

The first time a mother gets on her feet after giving birth, she may feel lightheaded. She might even faint. It is best for her to take things slowly, first sitting up, next dangling her feet over the side of the bed, then standing, and finally walking slowly and easily.

- If your partner wants to get up, have someone help. An experienced nurse can make these moves simple and easy. There is no rush. Take all the time she needs. The same step-by-step process applies to sitting up in the birthing chair after giving birth in it.

If your partner wants to empty her bladder, she may find it hard to let go at first. Nerves around the bladder take a while to return to normal. Tissues are tender and a little swollen. Pouring warm water over the perineum while she tries may bring success. Sitting on the toilet is more comfortable and natural than the bedpan. She may feel better leaning against you or a nurse for support.

Gently tightening and letting go with the muscles around her bladder and vagina (called the Kegal exercise) may help. Blood circulates more freely in muscles when they are used, carrying off fluids from swollen tissues and awakening nerve endings. Healing of the episiotomy can be speeded up the same way.

When the observation period is over, you will all **go to the maternity floor, or home** if that is your plan. Your partner may ride on a stretcher or a wheel chair to her room, or she may walk if she prefers to and the hospital allows it.

The baby may ride in her arms or in a special crib.

Many hospitals bring the new baby to the nursery at this time for 2 to 24 hours of further observation. Having mother and baby stay together in the mother's room (rooming in) starts afterwards.

In the nursery, **the baby will be weighed, measured, possibly bathed, and placed in a warm crib**.

- You and your partner may be invited to watch. If not, ask if you may.

   In some hospitals, mother and baby may stay together for the entire visit. In this case, all care of the baby is done in the mother's room.

After you accompany your partner to her room, you may stay for awhile, though some hospitals allow visitors only during visiting hours. At this point it is often hard for both of you to settle down. Your partner may feel tired but be too excited to sleep. And if the baby is in the nursery she may feel lonely. It is their first separation since the beginning, nine months ago.

- If you can stay for awhile, share your feelings together. A soothing backrub may feel wonderful to her.
- When you leave, ask whether you can bring her anything when you come back. Tell her where you will be and when you will return.
- Remind her that 4-point releasing will help her to rest.
- Stop at the nurses' desk and tell them how they can reach you.
- Find out when the baby will be brought to your partner and pass this information along to her.

You may come away from your experience with mixed feelings. Labor and birth are over. You might be ravenously hungry and enormously tired. At the same time, you can be on a high that lasts for days. You may feel in awe of the miracle of life recreated, and filled with pride and astonishment at the energy and endurance of your partner. You may look back on your experience as an ordeal, long and frightening. You may wonder if you were a good coach. You may feel close to the baby and to your partner, or you may feel like a stranger in a new world. When you get home, you may find the house lonely, or be glad for the peace and quiet.

- Let off some steam by sharing your news with people you care about. If there are other children at home, sit and talk with them awhile. Especially for those who are very young, the time you have been away is a mystery.

- Feed yourself. Get some sleep. Errands and chores can wait a few hours. Sipping a hot drink in bed may help you to unwind. Starting with your forehead, let go with every part of your body, all the way down to your feet. Rest well.

You deserve it.

□ □ □

"For me, labor without coaching would be, in the words of Simon and Garfunkel, 'an endless chain of cigarettes and magazines'. Me and Sammy Davis Jr. can both say we did it my way. I'm proud!"

"A husband who has not seen his wife in labor has not the haziest concept of the woman she is."

"My husband was rather negative through classes, but he was fantastic through this labor, and says he will help me through the next one."

"I had pictured birth as a means to an end, not the great, great experience it is in itself."

Quick Coaching Guide (After the Birth)

Remind yourself:

- You and your partner must keep hands off the sterile sheets.
- If it was prearranged, ask to cut the cord.
- If it was prearranged, ask to delay the eyedrops.

For an intrauterine exam:

- Encourage your partner in 4-point releasing.
- Coach her in the breathing of her choice.

For the stitching of an episiotomy:

- Encourage your partner in 4-point releasing and breathing.
- If necessary, encourage her to look at the baby and to talk with you.

When holding the baby:

- Keep all body parts covered except the face.
- Support the head and neck with one hand, the back and bottom with the other.

If the baby does not nurse:

- Remind your partner that this is normal. Sleepiness and disinterest will disappear.

For your partner to get out of bed:

- Wait for assistance.
- Use 4-point releasing.
- Go slowly.

Before you go home:

- If the baby is in the nursery, find out when he will first visit your partner.
- Tell your partner, and the nurses, where you will be and when you will return.
- Ask whether she needs anything from home.

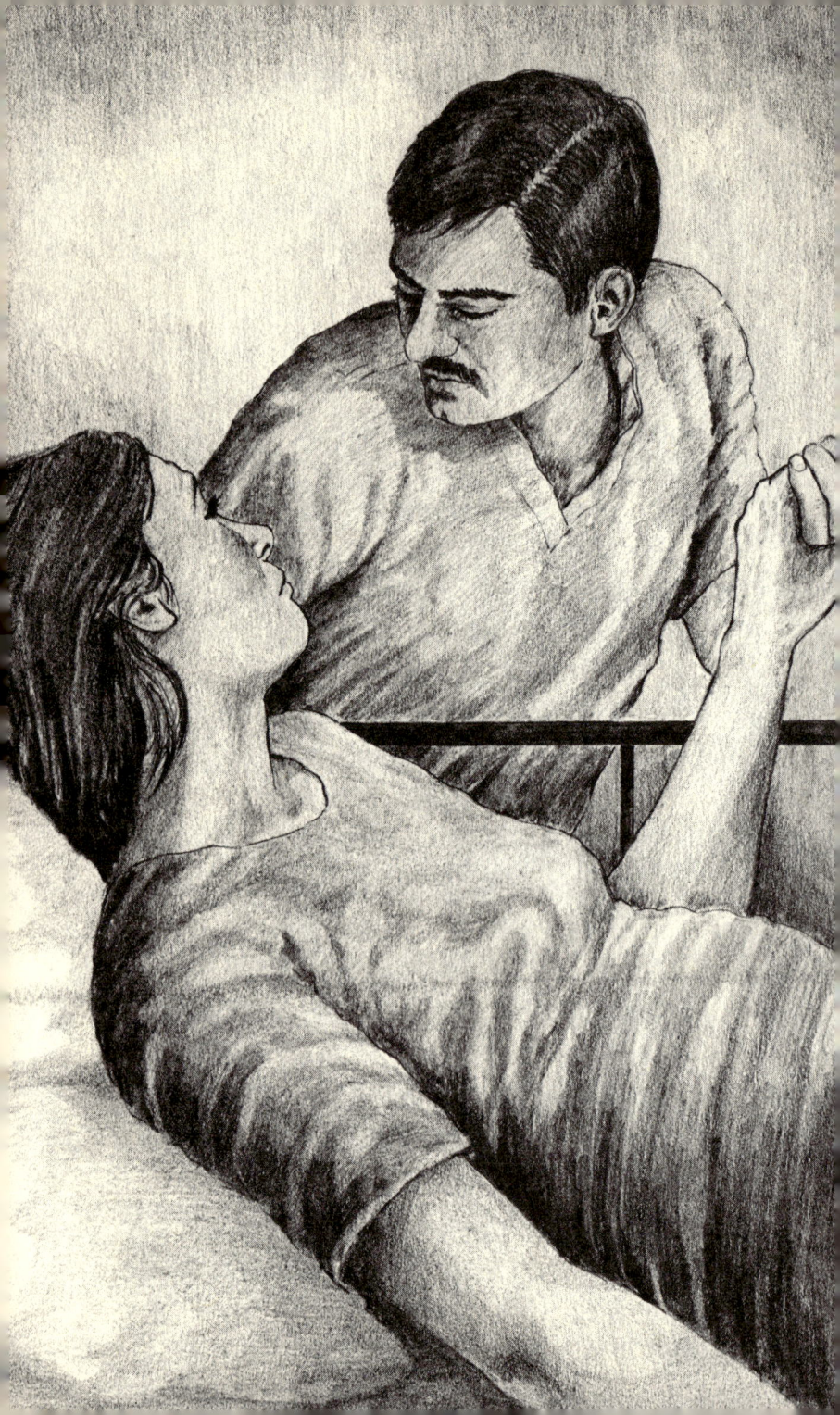

9. Coping with Pain

To speak of pain in labor is, of course, frightening. Often, classes and books avoid the subject, or mention it only briefly, perhaps substituting the word "discomfort"—out of concern about frightening women. Yet, after labor, women often say, "If I had only known it would hurt, I would have been prepared for it. Not expecting it—and then, surprised by its intensity—I thought something was going wrong."

This is the key. Although pain certainly is frightening to anticipate, it is easier to cope with if it is anticipated and if you prepare for it in advance.

How can we best handle pain? We fight pain because we don't like it, and because we are afraid of it. We tense up to fight pain, trying to protect ourselves against it. The problem is that we feel the pain anyway.

What happens if we relax when we are in pain, if we allow ourselves to feel the pain instead of trying to hold it at arm's length? When we relax, or let go of tension, we stop trying to fight off pain. We open ourselves to it instead. Surprisingly, the pain is not stronger once it is faced. It hurts about the same—but the pain centers in the area it is coming from (the uterus) instead of feeling as though it involves the entire body. The difference is that some of our fear is gone. No one is expected to like pain, but it is easier to cope with pain when we are not afraid of it.

This is not to say that with relaxation labor contractions become less powerful or that labor will be easy, even though a few women *do* find labor easy. Probably a woman is best prepared for labor if she accepts that she must do several hours of very hard work by herself. No one else can do the job for her. But she is not helpless. She has tools with which she can help herself. Information lets her anticipate what to expect. Relaxing and breathing help her to use energy constructively to work with her contractions. The encouragement, support, and suggestions of helpers strengthen her confidence. Cheered on, she can go farther. Cared about, she finds courage.

Attitude is important, for both the mother and the coach. For the mother, it usually helps to recognize that the pain of labor is different from the pain of illness or injury. In labor, she is moving toward something very positive, the arrival of a baby. It also is useful to understand that the pain comes from tissues that are stretching to open for the birth, that the body is functioning normally, as it is designed to do.

As the coach, it helps if you agree that it hurts. Because you care about your partner, you want to save her from hurt. You may be upset because you are helpless to do so. Out of frustration or guilt, you may be trying to play down pain—"It's not so bad, everybody lives through it." Medical attendants may say these things, too.

But denying or belittling pain only makes a woman feel guilty about her reactions, angry at being denied, and lonely because she is not understood. The pain she feels is very real, and emotions like fear and anger can intensify her perception of it.

You cannot stop the pain, but you *can* do a lot to help your partner cope with it. Recognizing that her emotions are a big part of her response, you will understand that comfort and relaxation can help to calm her. The idea is for her to work with her body without being hindered by negative reactions.

For you both, it is useful to think of the present moment as the only reality that needs attention and effort. Although you both remember contractions that have passed and worry about those to come, the fact is that you need work with only one contraction at a time. So think about only that one contraction. Take each one as it comes.

□ □ □

"I don't believe we were prepared for the intensity of the pain or maybe it was how fast it got intense. It was hard for me to get through to her with the breathing and relaxing."

"I was pretty scared and I sure felt sorry for myself, and some of the screaming was for attention or company."

"She always expressed her pain or frustration to me and the doctor, so it never welled up inside her in a destructive way."

"She felt if the pain was so great in the first stage, how could she possibly handle the next? We later found out she was in advanced labor while we were at home."

"I felt more pain when I severely sprained my ankle months before."

"Pain in labor is very real, not to be underrated. But by the next evening Julie could say, 'That wasn't so bad.' "

"I forgot how to breathe. Kevin looked right in my eyes, his head about 3 inches from mine, and said, 'Breathe with me.' It was like I had no choice. I lost my consciousness of what the doctor was doing and started my breathing."

□ □ □

The purpose of the skills a mother learns is to use them in order to work with labor, not to shut it out. Remember these basics:

- Use the cleansing breath to get into the contraction. Later, use another cleansing breath to let the contraction go.

- Use relaxing to go with the contraction, to stay calm, and to help keep breathing under control.

- Use breathings—and, later, pushing—to cooperate with the body's efforts.

- Between contractions, use nourishment and deep rest to keep up energy.

- Use intuition and experimentation to find positions that are as comfortable as possible, to help the mother to remain relaxed.

Quick Coaching Guide (Regaining Control)

Watch your partner to note and short-stop difficulties right away.

If you see **tension**, stress 4-point releasing.

If you see a **minor problem with breathing**—irregular, too fast, or deep when it should be shallow—try this:

- First, suggest 4-point releasing to break the cycle that is starting—pain = fear = tension = difficulty with breathing.

- Next, correct the breathing. Remember, breathing is deep and slow, or rapid and shallow. Continue to support what she is doing.

If **your partner loses control completely**, or is on the verge of doing so, try these steps:

1. Tell her to look at you. If her eyes are shut, you may need to tell her to "Open your eyes."

2. Next, have her breathe with you, copying you as you demonstrate: "Breathe with me."

3. Encourage her as she tries: "You can do it. Keep going."

4. Once you see that her breathing is somewhat under control, remind her of 4-point releasing.
5. Keep her looking at you, if control is shaky. Otherwise, she can gaze at her focal point.
6. Keep repeating reminders on how to release and how to breathe. You may have to be very firm.

The formula might go like this:

"Look at me."

"Breathe with me." (Demonstration) "Follow me."

"Keep going. Good."

"Now release your face, and now your shoulders."

"Keep breathing." (Demonstration)

"The contraction is over? Let it go with a big easy cleansing breath" (Demonstration)

"Now rest. I'll work with you on the next one. But for the present, just rest."

10. Born on the Way to the Hospital

"Because my first child was quite long in labor, I wasn't in a rush. Then suddenly I realized that we'd better hurry. Pete helped me to the car. I already had the urge to push."

□ □ □

You may have wondered what you would do if the baby arrived on the way to the hospital. It is possible, though unlikely. Most labors give enough advance warning, with contractions growing stronger and longer over a period of hours, to allow time for you and your partner to reach the hospital.

The following basic instructions will help if you are caught short (though they are *not* enough to handle a planned home delivery). When a baby slips so easily into the world that there is not time to get to the hospital, the helper's tasks are usually fairly simple. Actually, it is not so much a matter of knowing what to do as it is knowing what not to do.

When your partner feels the urge to push, make sure she does her no-push breathing. She will still feel the uterus bearing down and the baby moving through her vagina. But without her pushing help, the birth may be delayed until you reach the hospital. Because your partner avoids pushing, the baby will come out more slowly whenever he is born. The birth will be easier to manage and healthier for the child, and your partner's tissues are less likely to tear.

□ □ □

"I did everything I could not to push, but I knew the baby would come soon."

□ □ □

If you are within easy reach of a telephone, call your hospital. Tell the switchboard operator what is happening, that you and your partner are coming in, and that you want her to call your midwife or doctor. There will be medical attendants waiting to meet you when you arrive.

On the way to the hospital, avoid driving fast and wildly. Your partner will have greater difficulty staying in control if your driving makes her nervous. And an accident can be far more serious than a birth in the car. She needs your support. The physical and emotional feelings of giving birth are usually intense. You can add to your partner's confidence and to your own as well if you stay as calm as you can.

□ □ □

"When the moment comes to move fast, despite preparation there's that momentary fear, like the moment when you suddenly have the ball in your hands and you have to think clearly and make the right moves—but definitely more intense. I had never wanted anything so much as to see this baby safely delivered. It seems to me there are built-in instincts that come into play and help you do things you wouldn't expect."

□ □ □

If the baby starts to emerge, pull over to the side of the road and stop the car. Slow down if you can't stop.

Turn on your emergency flashers. If there is a telephone nearby and someone who can help, you could ask that an ambulance be called. But stay with your partner as much as possible, *especially* for the birth.

□ □ □

"She told me urgently to find a place to stop—the baby's head was already crowning—I felt the bump in her pants."

□ □ □

Your partner will be more comfortable on the back seat where she can more easily find a position to give the baby room to be born. There will be fluid—water from the uterus and blood from the cervix—so if possible, she should sit on something absorbent and as clean as you can find. Unread newspapers, or perhaps your coat (you can always take it to the cleaner's later) will do.

□ □ □

"I got in the back with her and slipped her pants down. She was in a good kneeling position."

□ □ □

Suggestion: Plan for the unexpected. About a month before the due date, put 2 or 3 large towels in your car, stored in a plastic bag to keep them clean. Although they probably will not be needed for a birth, they are useful to sit on if the water bag breaks before you reach the hospital. See page 72 for more about the breaking of the water bag.

It is not necessary to pull on the baby, cut the cord, wipe out the mouth, or try to remove the afterbirth. As he emerges, if the baby is still inside the water bag, tear it carefully *at the back of his head* with your fingernail or something else that is sharp. Lift the thin membrane of the bag away from the baby's face so he can breathe freely.

□ □ □

"There it was! Before I knew it, a little face had popped out. It all seemed so easy. A few air bubbles around the nose— breathing! No twisted cord on the neck."

□ □ □

Sometimes the cord is around a baby's neck. If this is the case, after he is born, very gently unwind it or lift it over his head.

Place the baby at a slant with his head lower than his body and his face down or to the side. This position will help to drain fluids from his nose and mouth.

Although this step is often unnecessary, you can use your fingers to stroke downward gently along the baby's nose, and upward along his throat in the direction of his chin, helping to remove liquids.

Almost all babies breathe on their own. Crying for a few minutes helps the baby to take in lots of oxygen. If he has not begun breathing within 30 to 45 seconds, he needs extra stimulation.

- Place 2 fingers on either side of his spine, above his buttocks, and run them up his back. Or briskly rub your hand up and down his back. Be firm but gentle.

- Keep him at a slant, with his head lower than his body.

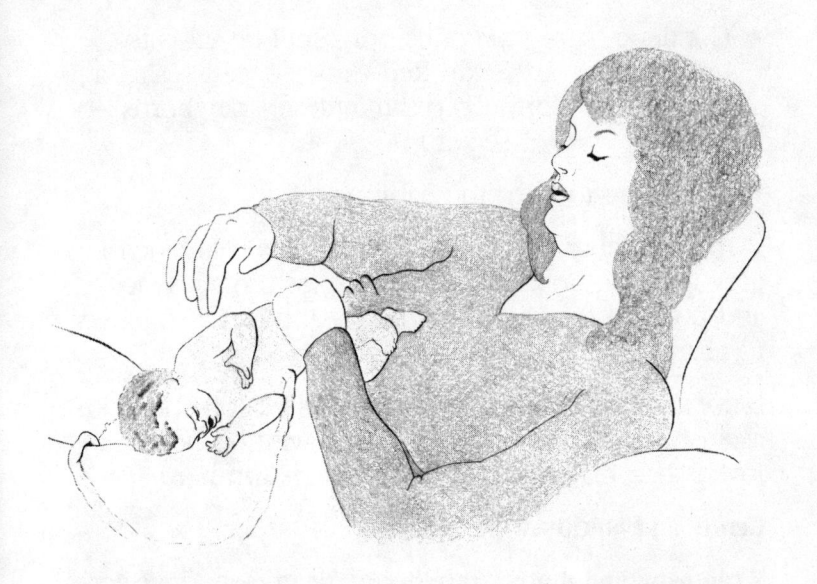

Place the baby at a slant.

Once in a rare while, in spite of this stimulation, a baby still will not breathe. If, at 60 seconds after birth, the baby is not breathing, take the next step. It must be done *very carefully* to avoid injuring the baby's delicate lungs.

- Gently tilt his head back a little so that his chin points upward.

- Place your mouth around both his mouth and nose.

- Four times, blow little puffs of air into his lungs. It is important that you **do NOT breathe deeply and then**

blow forcibly. Puff, gently, using the air from inside your mouth.

- Continue these little puffs only until he starts to breathe. The American Red Cross suggests using a rate of about 20 puffs per minute for newborns—or 1 breath every 3 seconds.
- Make sure to keep the baby warm.

Remember that a newborn baby is pale blue or grey in color, until his breathing transforms his face and body to rosy pink. His hands and feet take longer to change.

Leave the baby between your partner's legs or place him against her bare abdomen or chest with his head lower than his body. Her body will warm him.

Gently and quickly wipe him dry.

Wrap baby and mother together in clean coats, sweaters, towels, or blankets. Cover the baby's head, but leave his face exposed. Keep the baby warm. This is very important. The effort to keep himself warm uses the oxygen his body needs to adjust to life outside his mother.

□ □ □

"This was a good moment to sprint to the bus office nearby and tell an astonished ticket agent to call the hospital. It took less than 1 minute. When I got back Debbie was sitting like the Mother of God, holding the baby in a towel, with a truly beautiful and radiant smile on her face. She said, 'You have a boy.'"

Should the placenta come out before you reach the hospital, simply place it against the baby. It will act like a hot water bottle. Be sure to bring it to the hospital for your midwife or doctor to examine.

After it has emptied itself, the uterus must remain contracted to prevent excessive bleeding. It will do so by itself, although its contraction is helped along when:

1. The baby nurses (although some babies are not interested in nursing right after birth).
2. The mother's nipples are gently rolled and pulled between the fingers.

You or your partner can feel the uterus, which is now about the size of a large grapefruit, somewhere between your partner's navel and her pubic bone. If the uterus feels hard, it is contracted. If it feels soft, it is not contracted.

- If it is not contracted, and if the nipple stimulation does not work well enough, gently rub the top of the uterus through the abdominal wall to help it contract. Too much massage, though, can cause it to relax, so use this technique only when the uterus is soft, and only until it hardens. Your partner can also do this for herself.

Continue driving to the hospital.

□ □ □

"I was given a semi-private room and was able to nurse the baby in this room, but I felt somewhat isolated, and bored as well, because I wasn't tired, or sick."

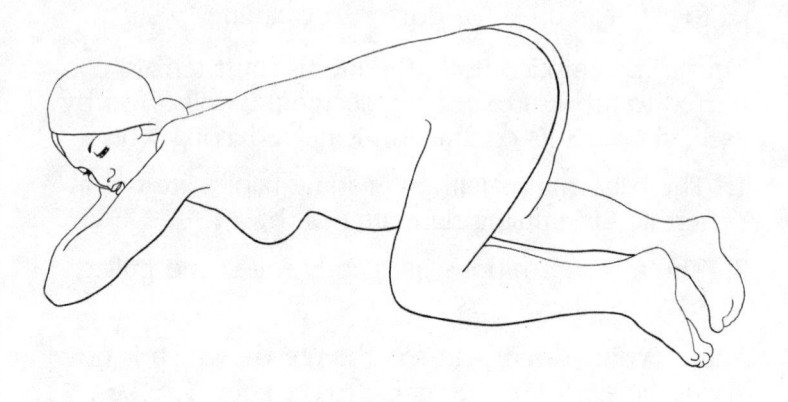

Knee-chest position.

Upon arriving at the hospital, babies born outside sometimes are put in rooms by themselves, in case they have picked up germs on the way in. Usually, mothers are not put in isolation. If your hospital has an unoccupied private room, mother and baby might be able to room together. This is medically acceptable, but visitors may be restricted.

A mother should be able to visit her baby if he is in isolation. Probably, she will have to wear a gown over her clothes while she is with the baby, and wash her hands before leaving. Usually a father will have the same freedom.

Rules like these depend on the written policies of your hospital. Speak to the head nurse on the maternity floor, or with your midwife or doctor, if there is a problem.

□ □ □

"We were able to take him home in 5 days. John Andrew is now a very strong and active 3-year-old with no health problems."

□ □ □

POSSIBLE PROBLEMS

Prolapsed cord:
When the water bag breaks, if you see a shiny blue-grey cord protruding from the vagina, this means that the umbilical cord, which normally remains above the baby's head in the uterus, has slipped down below it. This is called a *prolapsed cord*.

> **Your partner MUST remain in a knee-chest position. In this emergency the cord can be pinched between the baby and the mother's pelvis, cutting off oxygen to the baby. The knee-chest position helps to keep the baby above the pelvis, which may keep the pressure off the cord.**

If you are in the car:

- Help your partner into the knee-chest position (the car's back seat will be roomier) and loosely cover the cord with a soft clean cloth to keep it warm.

- **Keep going** to the emergency room entrance of your hospital.

- If your partner feels like pushing, **insist** that she do her no-push breathing.

Drive with care. This is a true emergency and you will be frightened, but an accident would make things much more difficult. Remain as calm as you can. You cannot perform miracles. You are doing your best.

If you are at home:

- **Place a warm, wet towel loosely around the cord.** The goal is to keep the cord warm and moist, but without pressure that could slow or stop its blood flow to the baby.

- **Telephone the hospital.** Tell the switchboard operator what has happened and that you are coming in. Ask her to call your doctor for you before she does anything else.

- **Telephone an ambulance.** Explain your situation and that you must reach the hospital quickly. The ambulance carries oxygen which, inhaled by your partner, may help the baby.

- If the ambulance will be delayed and if you feel competent to make the trip yourself, **go immediately to the emergency room entrance** of your hospital.

- **Drive with care.**

In this serious emergency, many babies do not survive. It is a difficult and tricky situation for anyone to handle—even the most able physician. If the outcome is an unhappy one, you must not blame yourselves, but know that you did everything possible under unusually demanding circumstances.

Remember that it is unlikely you will have any of

these experiences. Even so, it is best to know ahead of time what to do if they should occur.

For further information on emergency childbirth situations, please see *Further Reading* on page 299.

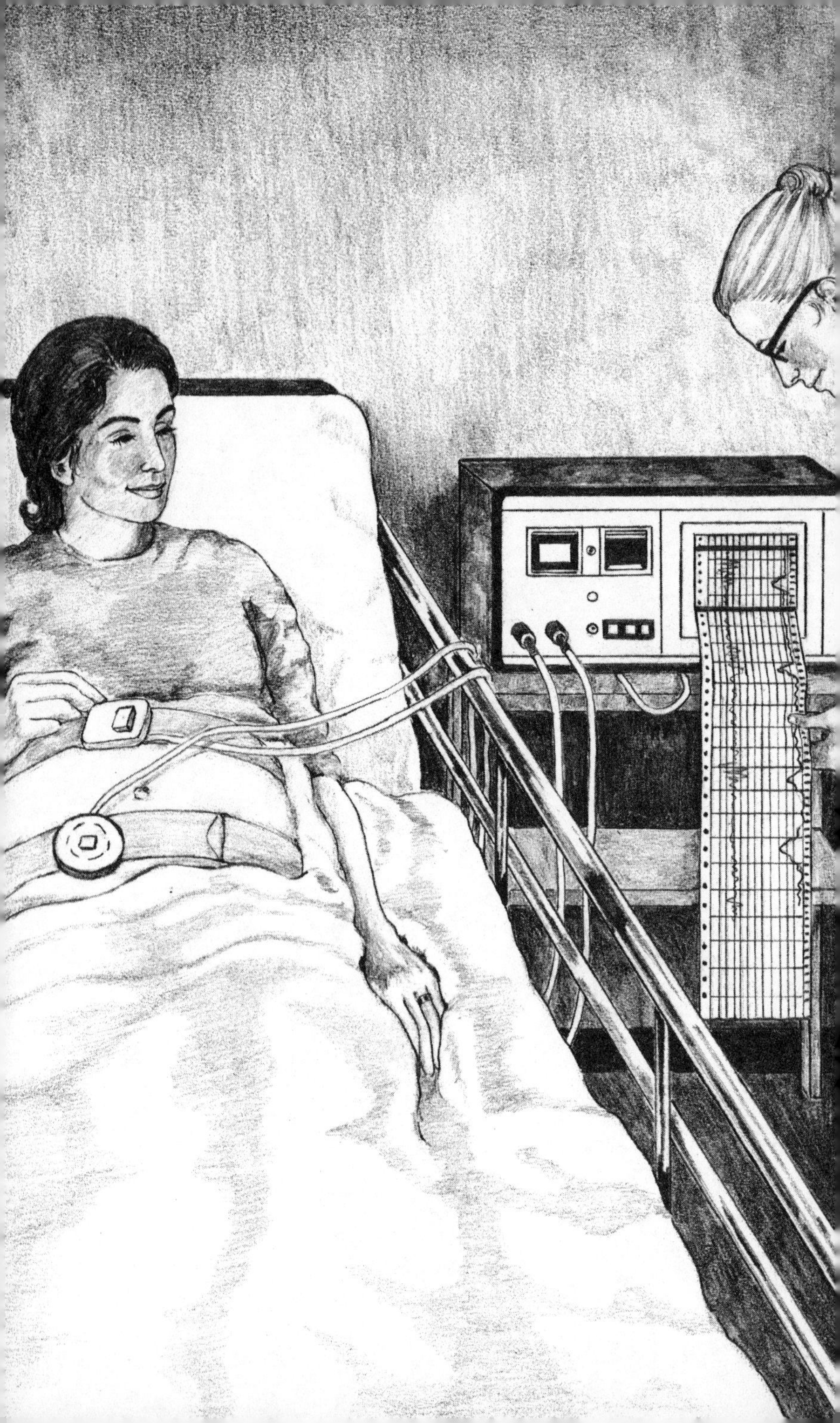

11. What to Expect with Hospital and Medical Procedures

Some of these hospital and medical procedures will be familiar to you and your partner. Some will not. You both can approach any of them more confidently if you understand them and know what to expect.

Here are a few details explaining how and why they are done. Which procedures may be used in your labor depends mostly on your midwife or doctor and, to some degree, on your hospital's policies.

Admission procedures take an average of about an hour. They may include:

UNDRESSING

When they enter the labor room, mothers are asked to undress and put on hospital gowns that tie in the back. A woman who is 9 months pregnant and in labor can have an awkward time getting out of her clothes.

- Your partner may be glad for your help as she changes into her gown. When a contraction comes, stop all activities, concentrate on 4-point releasing and, if it is being used by now, breathing.

VITAL SIGNS

Mother's blood pressure, pulse, breathing, and temperature, and baby's heartbeat all are checked on admission. To listen to the baby's heart, one of several types of fetoscopes is used. Like a stethoscope, the fetoscope picks up sounds from inside the body. A stethoscope transmits heart, lung, and bowel sounds. The more sensitive fetoscope makes it easier to hear the delicate beating of an unborn baby's heart.

- Ask the attendant if your partner and you can listen to the baby's heart. Hospital routines and the hard work of labor demand so much of your attention that the reality of the baby's birth can seem very far off. Hearing the heartbeat reminds you both of the reason for all your efforts.

URINALYSIS

Your partner will be shown to the bathroom and asked to urinate into a paper cup. Sometimes a bedpan placed in the toilet catches the urine, which the nurse transfers to a test tube. This specimen will be tested to show how your partner's kidneys are working and whether her body fluids are at a healthy level.

INTERNAL EXAMS

Vaginal (and sometimes rectal) exams are given on admission by a nurse, midwife, or doctor. From time to time throughout labor they are repeated, to check the cervix and the baby's head, which can be felt at the back of the vagina.

Exams may be given between contractions or

while a contraction is going on. During a contraction, the baby's head is pushed against the cervix, making it easier to get an accurate measurement of how much the cervix has flattened (effaced) and opened (dilated), and easier to measure the location of the baby's head within the mother's pelvis. Although some babies may slip back up during intervals, most remain in position, and exams made between contractions are nearly as accurate.

When the exam is done during a strong contraction, your partner may have to work hard to stay in control. You can help her.

- Talk your partner through 4-point releasing, emphasizing especially her bottom and thighs. Breathe with her, using her choice of breathing. Remind her to allow her body to remain open to the exam. This will help to make it go quickly.

- Ask the nurse, midwife, or doctor to tell you how much the cervix is effaced and dilated, and how far into the pelvis the baby has dropped. Have the attendant explain what this means about the progress of labor so that you know what to expect over the next few hours. If progress is slower than you had hoped, the facts can be discouraging, but knowing how things stand helps you both to ration your energy and pace yourselves.

PATIENT'S HISTORY

The nurse who admits your partner usually needs to fill out several forms requiring answers to many questions. Some are about past pregnancies, some about this pregnancy, and some about her health in general. Sometimes midwives or doctors who already have this information send it directly to the hospital several weeks before the baby is due.

- If your midwife or doctor does not send this information to the hospital, when you and your partner take the hospital tour in the last months of pregnancy, ask the person who shows you around if you may have a copy of the "patient's history form." Your partner can fill it out at home and bring it with her to the hospital when she is in labor. Regulations require that the nurse who admits your partner must fill out official forms herself, but she might be able to copy these basic facts and save your partner some time and energy.

The nurse will also want information on progress of labor so far.

- Before coming to the hospital, write down:
The time contractions first started;
How often they come and how long they last;
When the mucus plug or bloody show is first seen, how much there is, what its color is, and whether it continues;
When the water breaks and what it looks like;
Whether your partner has had bowel movements, sleep, food, and fluids, and how much of each.

SIGNING CONSENTS (PERMISSION FORMS)

Your partner may be asked to sign papers granting permission to her midwife or doctor to deliver her baby, and to the obstetrician to perform a circumcision if the baby is a boy (please read about circumcision on page 220), and giving permission to her pediatrician to care for the baby during the hospital stay. If your partner has not chosen a doctor for the baby, or if she prefers one who is not on the staff at the hospital where the baby will be born, the hospital pediatrician who is on call will be in charge while the baby is in the hospital. This same doctor can continue as the pediatrician after the baby is at home, or until another is chosen. It is a good idea to choose a pediatrician during the pregnancy, or at least before leaving the hospital, so that there will be a doctor to care for the baby outside the hospital.

BLOOD TESTS

Some doctors order blood tests to show, among other things, blood type, whether there are enough red blood cells to carry oxygen to mother and baby, and how quickly bleeding stops. A nurse or hospital attendant usually takes two samples.

SHAVE

Because clean hair carries no more germs than clean skin, it is rare these days for all the pubic hair to be shaved. A few doctors may still request a complete shave. Often, only the hair covering the labia and perineum is removed. Sometimes the shave is limited to the perineum if there is hair there, for performing and repairing the episiotomy. Many doctors merely clip away long hair or require no shave at all.

The soapy water used for the shave should be completely rinsed away. Otherwise the skin itches and stings. Most nurses are gentle though speedy.

- Before the nurse starts, you or your partner can ask her to go slowly and to stop during contractions.

- Should there be a reason why she can't wait, suggest to your partner that she concentrate as totally as possible on relaxing and breathing, if she is using it.

ENEMA

Some doctors require an enema to be given in labor to empty the bowels. Many of today's midwives and doctors bypass enemas because early labor contractions often stimulate bowel movements anyway, and it is easy to clean away any small bowel movements that may be passed while a mother is pushing during the second stage. While enemas also can make contractions stronger, today it is beginning to be recognized that nourishment, exercise, and the release of tension usually helps a woman's body to labor adequately without artificial stimulation.

If an enema is ordered, it usually is an SS enema (1 or 2 quarts of warm water and Soap Suds). Sometimes a Fleet Enema (a 4½ ounce tube of liquid chemical) is used instead. Of the two, the Fleet is more comfortable to receive. If you are with your partner when the enema is given, you can pass on some hints to help her stay in control.

- Before the nurse starts the enema, ask her to stop the flow of water during a contraction. It is easier to cope with the contraction and the water flow separately.

- To allow the tip of the enema tube to pass comfortably into her rectum, your partner can push out as for a bowel movement, thus opening up the ring of muscles around the anus.

- While she is receiving the enema, suggest that she release face, neck, shoulders, hands and feet continuously and take very slow, deep breaths. Count up to 12 or 16 breaths. By the time this number is reached, the enema will have been given and your partner will be on her way to the bathroom.

If you and your partner are at ease about remaining together while she is on the bedpan or in the bathroom, your presence can be reassuring. Bathrooms are lonely and often chilly. Sitting on bedpans or toilets is uncomfortable, and enema cramps combined with contractions can be hard to handle. If she is using a bedpan, sitting straight up usually feels more natural than lying down.

- The upper half of the bed can be raised to support her back while she squats or sits Indian style. Or she can place the bedpan on the edge of her bed and dangle her legs with a chair under her feet.

- You can sit on a chair next to her. She may relax more easily if she rests her head or body against you.

- Guide your partner in 4-point releasing. Remind her to breathe easily and slowly.

- You might suggest warm socks, a warm sweater around her shoulders, and a blanket across her knees.

- To safeguard against having to return to the toilet or bedpan, she will want to make sure she has passed all the enema. Suggest to her that she stay on the toilet or bedpan for a full 20 minutes, or, after she thinks she has finished, that she wait 5 more minutes.

IVs

An IV is fluid (usually glucose, a natural body sugar, and water) that flows from a bottle through a long, skinny tube, into a person's vein (*I*ntra-*V*enous). Some doctors order IVs for women during labor. This keeps the mother's body supplied with fluids, especially important if the doctor does not allow her to drink liquids during labor. The IV also provides an entrance to a vein for medications or blood if the midwife or doctor should order them. A needle is used to slip a very thin flexible tube into the vein. Only the tube, which has blunt, round ends, remains in the vein, held in place by adhesive tape, so that your partner can move about freely without fear of hurting herself or dislodging the IV. Occasionally, to safeguard the IV, the mother's hand or arm is taped to a slender, padded board.

The IV bottle is attached to a tall stand so the fluid can flow with the help of gravity. At the point where the IV tube passes into the mother's hand or arm, IV fluid sometimes enters (infiltrates) tissues instead of the vein. This causes the area around the IV tube to become puffy and to feel cold. If this happens, the IV is usually stopped and started at another spot. If the flow of IV fluid is interrupted (by a kink in the tube, or by the mother raising her arm too high, for example) blood from the vein with which the IV is connected will appear in the tubing. This is startling to see but usually can be remedied by a simple adjustment.

- If you notice this, or if you have any other questions about the IV, tell a nurse or your midwife or doctor right away.

THE FETAL MONITOR

The pattern on the graph paper of the fetal monitor as it charts the activity of the uterus looks like hills (contractions) and valleys (intervals). Read the graph by looking at it from the side.

- At the start of a contraction the line begins to travel uphill.
- When the contraction has passed its peak and starts to weaken, the line starts to travel downhill.
- When the contraction is over, the line flattens out until the beginning of the next contraction, when it starts uphill again.

> **Note**: This very sensitive machine also records the tightening of the abdomen for reasons other than contractions—coughs, hiccoughs, vomiting, pushing in the second stage, and so on. These show as extra peaks on the graph paper pattern of the working uterus.

The fetal monitor looks like a table-top stereo. The baby's heart rate and the mother's contractions are recorded on graph paper that rolls out slowly from the front of the machine, somewhat like tape from a wide cash register. This record shows how the baby's heart reacts to contractions. It also shows the length and strength of contractions. A baby's heart beats at an average rate of 120 to 160 beats per minute, about twice as fast as an adult's heart beats.

Two wide elastic straps are placed around the mother's body like belts. Where buckles would be, there are transmitters that pick up and send information through wires to the machine.

Instead of belts, some monitors use tiny recording units that pass through the vagina and attach to the baby's head, clipping onto or penetrating the outer skin of the baby's scalp. To use this device the water bag must have broken so the baby's head is exposed through the partly-open cervix. The wires coming from the vagina to the monitor are anchored to a strap placed around the mother's thigh. The advantage of the internal monitor is that the mother can move about freely within range of her link to the machine. The disadvantage is the possibility of infection or pain for the baby.

The newest internal monitoring models transmit information without using wires at all, giving the mother total freedom of movement.

The fetal monitor was designed originally to pass on extra information about the baby if problems are suspected during labor. For example, if the heart rhythm picked up with a fetoscope is irregular and needs to be checked further, or the doctor wants to watch the effect of artificially strengthened contractions on the baby in an induced or supplemented labor, a monitor might be used. Please read about induced labor on page 250.

Some doctors order the monitor on admission for all women. With this routine check, the monitor may be taken off after an hour or two or left on for the entire labor.

- If the monitor is used for your partner, ask to have the reasons explained.

So that information from external monitors is accurate, their placement on a mother's abdomen must be exact. The transmitter that records the baby's heartbeat (the transducer) is made slippery by the jelly placed on it to help pick up sounds. Because of this, the transmitter slides off target easily, so mothers usually are asked to remain in one position after it is placed.

Monitor belts need to be snug enough to keep the transducer in place, but not so tight that the mother is uncomfortable.

- Ask your partner how the belts feel. If they are too tight, don't hesitate to ask the nurse to loosen them.

Monitor belts interfere with a full abdomen massage, but if you use a little imagination it is still possible.

- Stroke from side to side between the belts or below the lower one. It may feel good to substitute a gentle massaging or stroking of shoulders, thighs, or back.

Often the machine senses the beginning of a contraction a moment before the mother does.

- When the graph paper shows you that a contraction is starting, encourage your partner to take her cleansing breath. A head start makes staying in control easier. During a particularly strong contraction your partner may be so busy concentrating on getting through it that she doesn't notice when it starts to let up.

- If you tell her when you see the change on the graph paper, she can tune in to her body instead of her effort, and ease her breathing to match the easing contraction.

- Ask a nurse to show you how to read the graph paper so that you can tell your partner when a contraction is coming, and when one is ending. Contractions and intervals look like mountains and valleys. The heartbeat is recorded as a long jagged line.

- If the volume control is turned up you may find it interesting and exciting to listen to the heartbeat. Sometimes, though, this or other sounds the machine makes may annoy your partner. The nurse can adjust the machine to eliminate all noises, so ask for assistance when you need it.

You might conclude that the monitor will be so useful to you in keeping track of contractions that you and your partner will ask to have it used. Have faith in your ability to cope with labor without it. As with all medical machines, it has disadvantages as well as advantages and should be used only when needed for medical reasons.

RUPTURING THE MEMBRANE

The water bag may break on its own at any time during labor. Or your midwife or doctor may break it when your partner is admitted to the hospital, or later on during labor. This simple procedure is done during a vaginal exam. The doctor can feel the water bag (membrane) bulging through the opening cervix like a balloon. He places a slender plastic tool that looks a little like a blunt crochet hook in the vagina and, guiding it with his fingers, makes a hole in the water bag. You will see anywhere from a small trickle to a large flow of clear or cloudy white water—the amniotic fluid. Read more about amniotic fluid on page 72.

During the procedure or immediately afterwards, a nurse listens to the baby's heart with a fetoscope, or fetal monitor. Because the water bag contains no nerves, there is no pain when it breaks. Your partner may find the vaginal exam uncomfortable, however. The change of pressure inside the uterus causes contractions to become stronger than they had been, either immediately or very soon. Your partner may be asked to stay in bed after the membrane is ruptured, using a bedpan for urinating.

- When the midwife or doctor ruptures the membrane, work with your partner as you do for a vaginal exam and for all contractions, reminding her to release point by point and to breathe easily and slowly.

Occasionally the water bag remains intact and surrounds the baby at birth.

EPISIOTOMY

The episiotomy is an incision made in a woman's perineum, the tissue between her vagina and her anus, at the time of giving birth. The cut can be made directly downward (a median incision) or off to one side (a medio-lateral incision). It is repaired with dissolvable stitches. Depending on the location and size of the cut, and on the tissues of the woman herself, healing can take from a few days to a month or so. Soreness, ranging from mild to severe, can last a couple of days or linger for several weeks.

The rationale supporting episiotomy is that:

1. It prevents tears and overstretch of vaginal tissue.
2. It allows the baby to be born sooner than would happen if the tissues were to take time to stretch to full capacity.

3. Enlarging the opening allows a baby in distress to be born quickly, or a large baby to be born more easily.

The episiotomy is made after the baby has been pushed by the mother and her uterus down to the vaginal opening. The pressure of the baby against the perineum causes it to become numb, and the midwife or doctor adds an injection of medication similar to novocaine. (Please read about medications on page 221).

The rationale that opposes episiotomy argues that:

1. It is medically unnecessary except for a certain percentage of women, although it is almost always done in the United States for first-time mothers (and somewhat less frequently for women having subsequent babies).

2. Good vaginal muscle tone reduces and corrects stretching that occurs during birth. Good tone can be achieved and maintained with exercise—tightening the perineal muscles as though holding back urine, and then releasing them, at least 50 times daily (the Kegal exercise).

3. For delivery, perineal massage, hot compresses, positioning (legs only moderately separated by delivery table stirrups) to allow flexibility of perineal tissue, and gentle pushing all permit the perineum to stretch without tears, or with small ones that are simple to repair.

Talk with your midwife or doctor and childbirth teacher to exchange opinions on episiotomies, and to gain more information. Also see *Further Reading* on page 299.

LEBOYER BATH

The Leboyer method pays special attention to the baby's feelings at birth and during the time immediately afterward. Inside the mother the baby experiences darkness, subdued sounds, a degree of weightlessness, continuous warmth, and a close physical environment. Birth causes some dramatic changes.

Many people believe that the baby should be given special attention during this transition. This includes having lights turned low during and after delivery, and having all sound—including voices—quiet. The baby is handled gently and sometimes given a slow, soothing massage immediately after birth. Within the first hour after birth the father, or other person with a special relationship with the baby, bathes the baby. This isn't a scrub-and-clean-up bath, but floating in warm water while being held securely. After the bath, the baby is dried thoroughly and kept warm.

"Bonding," or establishing first emotional ties with the parents, by being cuddled and talked to by the parents, with eye contact if the baby's eyes are open, is not specifically Leboyer but is recognized as an important step.

Several weeks before the baby is due to be born, find out your doctor's views on the Leboyer method, and discuss any special wishes of yours with him or her, so that you can arrange the birth as you would like it.

SILVER NITRATE MEDICATION

Most states in the United States have laws requiring that silver nitrate drops be placed in all babies' eyes at birth. This is to prevent eye infection from contact with gonorrhea bacteria, should they be present in the mother's vagina.

Silver nitrate can cause redness, swelling, and discharge that is temporary, lasting for a few days. Some states permit the use of other medications that are less irritating, usually tetracycline or erythromycin ointments.

Many babies shut their eyes in reaction to the medications and, for all, vision is temporarily blurred. If you and your partner want to make eye contact with your baby at birth, you may ask that these medications be delayed. A delay of up to an hour does not change their effectiveness.

CIRCUMCISION

Circumcision is the cutting away of the loose skin (foreskin) that covers the head of the penis. It is done by the obstetrician, usually when the baby is 2 or 3 days old, and sometimes within an hour or so after birth. Jews circumcize on the eighth day. The longer wait gives the baby more time to adjust to life outside the mother.

Circumcision is most popular in the United States where, at the beginning of this century, doctors believed it prevented cancer and venereal disease. This has since been disproved. The American Academy of Pediatricians states that there is no medical reason for circumcision. Circumcision continues to be done in the United States for religious reasons or because it is traditional. The foreskin normally is not retractable at birth. It loosens over a period of time until it can be pulled back fully for most boys by age 3.

When properly done, circumcision is safe. As

with any operation, there are possible side effects. Before the operation may be done, a signed permission form is required from the baby's mother.

For parents, the best way to reach a satisfactory decision about whether or not to circumcise is to collect the facts and then make up their minds. Talk with your obstetrician and pediatrician. You can also add to your understanding from reading. Please see *Further Reading,* on page 299.

MEDICATIONS DURING LABOR

Parents ask many questions about medications during labor. Are they safe for mother and baby? Will taking them mean labor wasn't "natural," that the mother failed? Will they impede awareness and/or ability to concentrate? What are the side effects?

Medications for labor can be best understood if they are divided into four groups. **Tranquilizers and sedatives** relieve anxiety and encourage rest. **Analgesics** relieve pain and are different from **anesthetics**, which remove all feeling. **Synthetic hormones** stimulate contractions. Any one drug may be given in amounts varying from small to medium to large, but in general all medications are used sparingly to minimize effects on the baby.

Tranquilizers or sedatives may be suggested in early labor to help in relieving anxiety or tension or to help a mother sleep for a while. Well-rehearsed relaxation and a philosophy of being open to labor instead of working against it, plus comfortable surroundings with loving support, are remarkably effective in achieving the same results or in helping the medication to work well.

Analgesics to ease the pain of contractions generally are given only after labor is well underway because they tend to slow or stop early mild contractions.

Local anesthetics numb a specific area, such as the mother's perineum for an episiotomy. Directly before birth, pressure from the baby against the perineum also numbs it. After birth, the medication is especially useful during stitching, when the body's natural anesthesia has worn off. Spinals are also local anesthesia. They numb the body below the point at which they are given and are used for births, during the use of forceps, and for Cesareans. Mothers may wonder about problems that might be caused by spinals. When they are given by an experienced, skillful doctor, they are unlikely to cause harmful side effects. In China, acupuncture is well known as a local anesthesia, but it is not commonly used in the United States.

General anesthesia may be used instead of local anesthesia during births, the use of forceps, and Cesareans.

A **synthetic hormone** often is given to the mother directly after her baby's birth. It helps the uterus to push out the afterbirth and then to remain contracted to lessen bleeding. The baby's nursing has the same effect, although not all babies are eager to nurse as soon as they are born.

A synthetic hormone is sometimes used to start labor contractions when the breaking of the water bag is not followed by contractions within a few hours. This is called inducing labor, or induction (for details on induction, see page 250). A synthetic hormone also can be given to strengthen contractions when they are thought to be too ineffective to advance labor. This is called supplementing labor. The mother can often solve the problem of weak contractions herself in the same way she copes with pain, plus

1. Releasing tension with 4-point releasing.
2. Remaining active in labor rather than lying in bed without moving for hours.
3. Using upright positions to allow gravity to help the baby move down and out of her body.

Please read about induced and supplemented labor on page 250 for more details.

All medications taken by a mother travel through her blood to her placenta, where they continue on to her baby. Rather than asking whether a drug reaches the baby, to which the answer is always "yes," we should ask first what effect(s) it has. Second, we need to ask whether the effect will be a problem. This depends on:

1. The amount of drug given.
2. When, in labor, it is given.

For example, a drug may not cause trouble for an unborn baby, but it might cause trouble after the baby is born. It is important to remember that medications affect each woman a little differently, and that the effect is lesser or greater according to the amount given.

The main concern of a midwife or doctor is to manage labor so as to ensure the well-being of mother and child. Ideally, medication is used only when nature's best efforts, usually dependable, need a hand.

MEDICINES AND DRUGS

Here is a list of medications commonly used during labor and birth. You and your partner might bring it with you to an appointment with your midwife or doctor so that you can talk together about those you may be offered. Most midwives and doctors have narrowed their choices to a few that they know and like especially well.

Only basic information is included. For greater detail, read the *Physicians' Desk Reference* (known as the *PDR*), a huge encyclopedia on drugs, available in every midwife's and doctor's office, in all pharmacies, and in some bookstores. A simpler and shorter reference is the *Medication Chart* by Betsy K. Adrian and Nada Logan Stotland (American Society for Psychoprophylaxis in Obstetrics; see page 300 for the address).

SEDATIVES soothe and calm.

Examples: Nembutal, Seconal, Tuinal.

Why given: For sleep in early labor; for rest between contractions and to lessen nervousness in active labor.

When given: In first stage of labor.

How given: By mouth (pill); by injection into a muscle in an arm or buttock (IM); by injection into a vein (IV), usually in an arm or hand.

Effects on baby: Given in large doses close to birth, may cause newborn to be sleepy, and to have difficulty with breathing, sucking.

Effects on mother: Large amounts may cause sleepiness and confusion.

Effect on labor: May slow a premature labor if given in large amounts.

TRANQUILIZERS soothe and calm.

Examples: Largon, Phenergan, Valium, Vistaril.

Why given: For calmness; to stop nausea.

When given: In first stage of labor.

How given: Same as sedatives.

Effects on baby: In large doses, may slow down the central nervous system; Valium, especially, affects the baby in many ways.

Effects on mother: May cause sleepiness; strengthens the effects of sedatives and analgesics, so smaller doses of these can be given.

Effect on labor: None known.

ANALGESICS lessen pain.

Examples: Demerol, morphine, Nisentil.

Why given: To lessen pain of contractions; to lessen nervousness; to help physical relaxation.

When given: During active labor, first stage.

How given: By injection into a muscle (IM) in an arm or buttock; by injection into a vein (IV), usually in an arm or hand.

Effects on baby: When given close to birth, may slow down many functions of newly-born baby.

Effects on mother: If mother becomes too sleepy, she may find it hard to wake up enough to work with her contractions.

Effect on labor: In early labor, can slow contractions; can keep uterus and mother from working with full energy in second stage, leading to use of forceps.

AMNESICS cause amnesia (forgetfulness).

Examples: Scopolamine (given with Demerol).

Why given: To take away the memory of pain and of labor.

When given: During active labor, first stage.

How given: Same as analgesics.

Effects on baby: Slight slow-down in body functions.

Effects on mother: Causes agitation, noisiness, hallucinations (imagining things that are not real); may leave mother partly aware during and after birth, feeling out of control and unable to work with labor.

Effect on labor: Because mother cannot work with her body, second stage may be longer, leading to use of forceps.

PITOCIN causes uterus to contract.

Other examples: Oxytocin, Syntocinon.

Why given: To start labor (induction) or to strengthen contractions.

When given: First or second stage.

How given: By injection into vein (IV) for first or second stage; IV or injection into muscle (IM) in third stage.

Effects on baby: If mother's blood pressure drops, baby's oxygen supply drops and heart rate may slow; connected with rise in jaundice (bilirubin) after birth.

Effects on mother: Blood pressure may drop; heart rate may become irregular.

Effect on labor: Causes strong contractions with short intervals.

INTRAVENOUS FLUIDS

Examples: Sterilized, distilled water mixed with glucose, saline, or other substances.

Why given: To maintain normal fluid level; to provide a means by which to give medications or blood; to help raise blood pressure if necessary.

When given: In any of the three stages.

How given: By injection into vein (IV), usually in arm or hand.

Effects on baby: No negative effects when IVs are properly inserted.

Effects on mother: Needs to urinate more often; possible infiltration of IV fluid into body tissue where needle has been inserted or backup of blood into tubing.

Effect on labor: No negative effect.

PARACERVICAL BLOCK blocks nerves in and around (para) the cervix.

Examples: "Caine" drugs such as novocaine, lidocaine, procaine, xylocaine.

Why given: To numb the cervix (the main source of pain from contractions) and the lower part of the uterus; lasts from 30 minutes to 2 hours.

When given: In first stage, after cervix is dilated between 4 and 9 centimeters.

How given: By injection into the uterus on either side of the cervix.

Effects on baby: Can slow baby's heart rate; during labor, fetal monitor may be used to check on this.

Effects on mother: Sometimes drug has no effect or numbs only part of the cervix; not to be used if mother is allergic to "caine" drugs.

Effect on labor: When first given, can slow contractions for awhile.

CAUDAL and EPIDURAL anesthesias remove all pain (and other feeling) from navel to toes.

Examples: "Caine" drugs—novocaine, lidocaine, procaine, xylocaine.

When given: During active labor in the first stage, or shortly before birth.

How given: Single injection into a space at the lower tip of the spine (Caudal) or between 2 vertebrae (back bones) low on the back (Epidural), outside the spinal canal which contains the spinal fluid; continuous flow of medication over a period of 15 to 45 minutes (thin tube replaces the injection needle, is held in place by tape).

Effects on baby: If mother's blood pressure drops, baby's oxygen supply drops and heart rate may slow.

Effects on mother: Blood pressure may drop; may have backache after birth; until medication wears off, can't move legs (up to 2 hours after birth). Not to be used if mother is allergic to "caine" drugs.

Effect on labor: Contractions may be less efficient, causing longer labor and help with forceps at birth; mother may have no feeling to push.

SADDLE BLOCK takes away all feeling from perineum, lower buttocks, and inner thighs (body parts that touch a saddle on a horse); usually used for vaginal birth only.

Examples: Same as Caudal.

When given: Given shortly before birth.

How given: After skin is numbed with a small injection, a single injection of anesthesia is given between 2 vertebrae a little higher on the back than for the epidural; enters spinal canal (fluid-filled canal around spinal cord); takes 5 to 10 minutes to give, has an effect within seconds.

Effects on baby: May slow working of central nervous system; if mother's blood pressure drops, baby's oxygen supply drops and heart rate may slow.

Effects on mother: Mother is awake and alert; may feel tugging if forceps are used; blood pressure may drop; after birth she should lie flat (though she can move) for 6 to 8 hours and drink lots of fluids to prevent headaches; numbness wears off in up to 2 hours.

Effect on labor: Because mother has no feeling to push, forceps may be used for the birth.

SPINAL takes away all feeling from just under the breasts down to the toes. Usually used for Cesarean birth.

Examples: Same as Caudal.

When given: Same as Saddle Block.

How given: Injection of anesthesia between 2 vertebrae a little higher on the back than for Saddle Block; enters spinal canal.

Effects on baby: Same as Saddle Block.

Effects on mother: May feel nausea, need for air (due to drug's effect on lower breathing muscles); may feel tugging during Cesarean; occasionally anesthesia is not totally effective; otherwise same as Saddle Block.

Effect on labor: Same as Saddle Block.

GENERAL ANESTHESIA causes overall or total loss of consciousness.

Examples: Gas, such as ether or nitrous oxide; sodium pentathol.

When given: Given immediately before birth or Cesarean, in order to affect the baby as little as possible.

How given: Gas is inhaled through a rubber mask placed over nose and mouth; sodium pentathol is received through an IV.

Effects on baby: Affects baby many ways, particularly causing sleepiness and difficulty with breathing.

Effects on mother: Mother is totally unaware if anesthesia is given steadily; she drifts between being asleep and awake if anesthesia is given on and off. Especially with gas, mother may vomit as she awakens; mother may not remember early minutes after awakening.

Effect on labor: Because contractions are less strong, forceps may be used with a vaginal birth; the uterus may bleed more than usual after birth because it contracts less strongly.

LOCAL (or regional) ANESTHESIA causes numbing of a certain area.

Examples: Same as Caudal.

Why given: To numb the perineum for an episiotomy done just before birth, and its repair (stitching) done just after birth.

When given: Just before the episiotomy; may be repeated during stitching if the mother is in pain.

How given: Injected into the perineum; this is felt little or not at all because perineum is already becoming numb from pressure of the baby's head in the vagina.

Effects on baby: Usually none is apparent.

Effects on mother: Usually none is apparent; may take

a few minutes to work; not to be used by mothers who are allergic to "caine" drugs.

Effect on labor: None.

PUDENDAL BLOCK numbs pudendal nerves in the vagina.

Examples: Same as Caudal.

Why given: To numb a greater area of the perineum than local anesthesia reaches, and the vagina as well.

When given: Within 30 minutes or less before birth.

How given: Injected inside the vagina or through the perineum.

Effects on baby: Same as Local.

Effects on mother: Same as Local.

Effect on labor: Same as Local.

TRILENE MASK: Cylinder (like a small flashlight) with rubber mask at one end.

Examples: Gas, such as Trilene, Penthrane.

Why given: To lessen pain with some lessening of consciousness but usually without putting mother to sleep.

When given: During contractions only, in last part of labor's first stage, and in second stage.

How given: Mask is attached to container held by mother; as she needs relief she holds mask over her nose and mouth and inhales; effective within 2-3 minutes.

Effects on baby: May cause difficulty with breathing for newborn.

Effects on mother: Possible vomiting, difficulties with breathing; must be used only when trained professionals are present.

Effect on labor: None known.

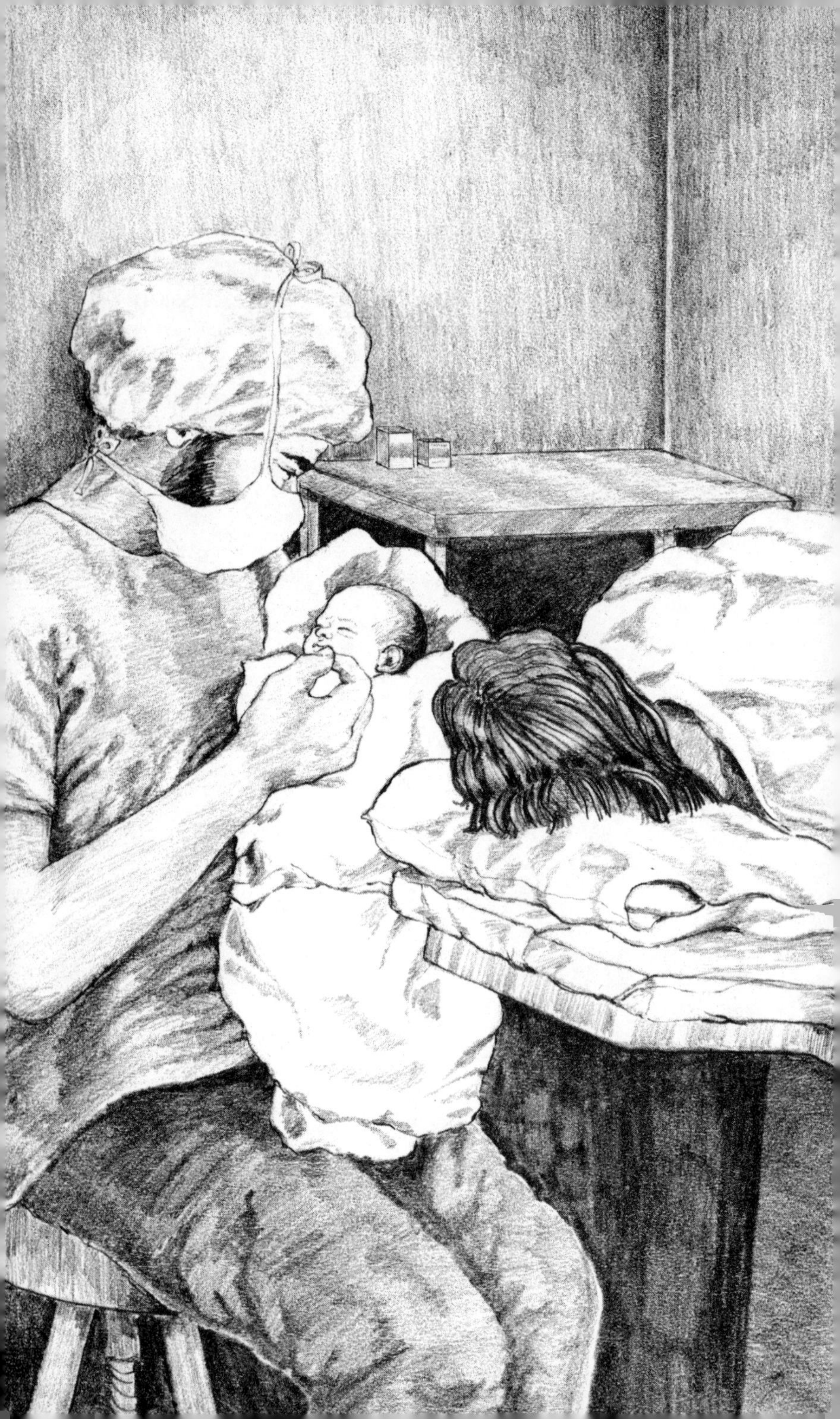

12. What to Expect with Variations in Labor

Although a few women have textbook labors, the majority encounter a few surprises, some small, some big. Although you and your partner may meet none of these variations, it is best to know your way around, and to know what your midwife or doctor might do in response to some common variations, just in case.

HYPERVENTILATION

Hyperventilation means that there is too much (*hyper*) oxygen (*ventilation*) and too little carbon dioxide in a person's system. Hyperventilation sneaks up on you. It comes from breathing that is *both* fast and deep.

> **To avoid hyperventilation** in labor, remember:
> **Deep** breathing must be **slow** breathing.
> **Rapid** breathing must be **shallow** breathing.

Tension or strong contractions make it easy for your partner to slip into breathing that is fast and deep.

Your first warning may be when your partner says she feels dizzy, numb around her mouth, tingly in her hands, or nauseated—all signs of hyperventilation. Or, as you watch her breathe with contractions, you may see that her breathing is both fast and deep, and you may suspect the onset of hyperventilation.

- When the contraction is over, tell your partner what you have observed. Ask her if she feels any of the symptoms of hyperventilation. If she says "yes," you know for certain that her breathing needs to be altered. If she says "no," wait through 2 or 3 more contractions to see whether symptoms develop. You may be overcautious, but check again soon.

Your task is twofold. First, adjust the breathing; second, get rid of the symptoms.

To adjust your partner's breathing:

- Watch your partner's breathing carefully with her next contraction. *Slow deep breathing*, if this is what she is using, means 9 or fewer breaths per minute, not counting the 2 cleansing breaths.

- Rather than telling her to "slow down your breathing," you will get the best results if you explain exactly how to breathe. At the same time demonstrate, telling her to breathe with you.

- Remind her to breathe in gently, without effort, to let herself fill up with air.

- As she exhales, she should blow out like a gentle, silent whistle. Suggest that she imagine she is making a candle flame flicker slightly, or sending a feather slowly through the air.

- As you breathe with her, raise your hand slowly as you inhale, lower it slowly as you exhale. Women often find it easier to adjust the pace of their breathing to hand movements.

- If your partner is using one of the *rapid and shallow breathings*, each inhalation and exhalation should be kept equal in length. The pace should be even. Eight or 10 breaths in a 5 second period is a workable rate.

- Use short up-and-down movements of your arm, or even a finger, to lead your partner, as if you were conducting an orchestra—up for inhalation, down for exhalation. Mark a 4/4 or a 2/4 beat, as in music. Emphasize the downbeat: ONE-two-three-four, ONE-two-three-four, or ONE-two, ONE-two.

- If she is breathing too fast, tell her: "I think you may be too fast. Try to follow me, as I breathe a little more slowly." After she has slowed down, set yourself to her pace rather than to your own.

- One trick is to sing or hum lightly with each exhalation. This allows her to be more aware of how she is breathing, and also automatically makes the breathing come out correctly. Follow a gently staccato rhythm. Make sure she keeps the breathing shallow.

- As she works, remind her of 4-point releasing with every breath. Tension always interferes with proper breathing.

- Between contractions, talk about your teamwork to make sure you understand each other.

To rebalance the oxygen and carbon dioxide in her blood, which will rid her of the symptoms of hyperventilation:

- If she breathes slowly and deeply into a small paper bag (the right size is about 4 inches wide by 7 inches long) or into her hands cupped around her nose and mouth, she will inhale some of the carbon dioxide that she exhales. This will raise the amount of carbon dioxide in her blood. This is easiest to do between contractions. If hyperventilation is severe, or contractions are so strong that it is difficult for your partner to keep her contraction breathing smooth and even, she can do her contraction breathing, too, into the paper bag or her cupped hands.

- Holding her breath will lower the oxygen, but because this creates tension, it is not advisable—unless she is about to begin pushing. When pushing starts, holding her breath is often normal for a woman.

- If she prefers to concentrate on relaxing and breathing, you can substitute your cupped hands in front of her face, about 5 inches away. She is likely to feel claustrophobic when hands other than her own are directly against her face.

- Do this until all signs of hyperventilation disappear or as long as contraction breathing is likely to cause hyperventilation.

FORCEPS

The idea of using forceps to help a baby to be born frightens many parents. In fact, when they are used by a skillful doctor with careful judgment there is very little chance of injury to mother or baby.

Forceps may be used at the end of labor's second stage if the mother's natural body forces need help to complete the birth. Common reasons might be:

- A tight fit between baby and pelvis

- A very tired mother or uterus
- A mother who should not strain herself with pushing because of a medical problem such as heart trouble or asthma
- A baby whose heart rate suddenly drops (indicating distress), so that it would be best for the baby to be born quickly
- A baby who has not turned into a position that will allow passage through the pelvis

Should such problems occur in the first stage of labor, when the baby is high in the pelvis, a Cesarean would be performed instead of using forceps. Forceps are used only when the baby is well down in the vagina ready to be born.

Forceps look like 2 very large spoons made of stainless steel with a hole in the bowl of each spoon. The bowls—or blades, as they are called—are curved to fit the sides of a baby's head and the mother's birth canal.

They are put in place during a rest period between contractions. One at a time is slipped into the vagina to rest alongside the baby's head. Once both forceps are in place, they connect to each other outside the mother, just above the blades, where the handles begin. This ensures that they will stay in the correct position.

The doctor uses the forceps during contractions only, working closely with the natural forces of the woman's body. Imitating nature, he uses the same amount of power as he pulls that the mother and uterus use as they push, while guiding the baby to follow the birth canal's natural curves.

As soon as the baby moves to the desired point,

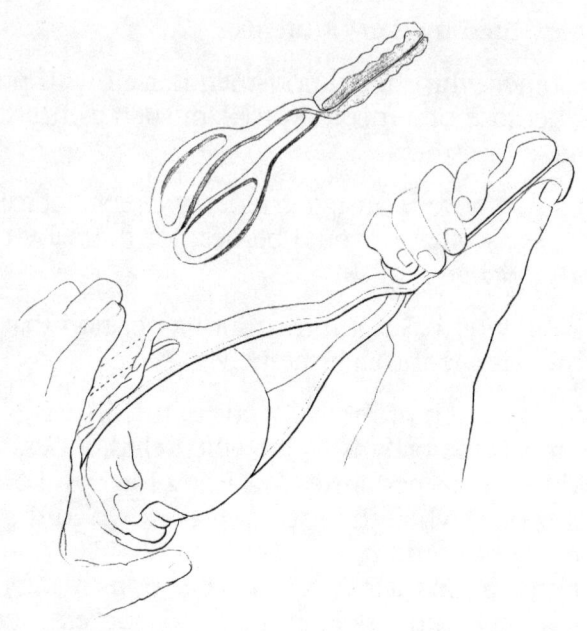

Forceps in place

the forceps are removed and the baby is born by the natural efforts of the mother and her uterus. While the forceps are in use—usually a minute or less—some mothers say that they feel intense pressure or pulling; others feel pain, too. Some doctors use spinal or general anesthesia with forceps, and some do not.

You may be asked to leave or permitted to stay. If you are present, it is understandable if you worry about your partner and the baby when you see how strong a force the doctor uses.

- Your best bet is to build up some trust in your doctor ahead of time by talking together at an office visit about this possibility.

- If you are using a midwife, ask whether she will call in an obstetrician should forceps be necessary.

If your partner does not have anesthesia, she can assist herself a lot by pushing strongly during contractions while the forceps are being used. You can help her to stay in control and to work with her contraction and the doctor.

- Talk to her as she pushes. Encourage her to go with the pushing urge, to open her body, to push strongly and long. Remind her that what she feels is not causing her harm, although the sensations are strong and even painful. Remind her to *push through pain*. Encourage her to work with the moment, which will last only as long as the contraction, about 60 seconds—just one minute.

When forceps are used skillfully, they are a wonderful tool to help transform a potentially serious problem into a safe delivery.

X-RAYS

X-rays may be ordered if your doctor wants to know the exact size and shape of your partner's pelvis and the exact size and position of the baby. These measurements have been checked in office visits, but in labor slight differences may appear that could not be detected by manual examination. During pregnancy, x-rays and sonograms are not taken routinely because of possible effects on the baby's development (proven to be damageable by x-rays; effects are still unknown with sonograms). Once the baby is ready to be born, x-rays do not seem to cause further damage to development, and a detailed photograph can help the doctor to decide whether a Cesarean may be the safest method of birth.

In most hospitals, the x-ray department is an elevator ride away, on another floor. Mothers are taken in their beds or on stretchers, by wheelchair or on foot. Your presence is as important now as at any time in labor.

- The ride may be uncomfortable. If your partner uses a bed or stretcher, you can help her to find the position that feels best. She may be happier on her side, even though the stretcher is narrow. If she remains on her back, at least 2 pillows should support her head and shoulders so that she is not completely flat. If she is more comfortable with her knees bent, raised side rails on the bed or stretcher give her legs something to rest against.

- Bring anything you have been using for her comfort (Chapstick, wet washcloths, and so on).

- Watch her arms, hands, and feet to make sure they aren't bumped as you pass through narrow doorways.

- Having an elevator to yourselves gives you more privacy. You can ask the nurse with you to request visitors to step out and wait for the next car. Hospital personnel, however, may ride with you.

- This change in your routine will make concentration more difficult. Each time your partner has a contraction, ignore everything and everybody but her. Except for emergencies, anything that was about to be done can wait for the short time one contraction lasts (except an empty elevator—better grab that!). Talk to your partner as you would in the labor room. Guide and encourage her with breathing. Remind her of 4-point releasing during contractions and between them. Holding her hand or touching her shoulder reassures her, especially if there is a lot of hustle and bustle going on around you, or if your attention is sidetracked for a moment.

In the x-ray room your partner will be asked to move to the hard surface of the x-ray table. Padding (the thin stretcher mattress, for example) placed on the table will make your partner more comfortable. The padding can cause a slight magnification on pictures that would have to be taken into account when they are interpreted. Because of this, the x-ray technician may decide against allowing the use of padding.

Several shots will be taken. Everyone leaves the room for each shot, only a few seconds.

- The x-ray technician will ask your partner to hold her breath while each picture is taken. Remind him that she needs to breath with contractions. He can time the picture-taking for intervals.

At times, coaches are asked to wait outside the x-ray room for the entire proceeding.

- Explain to those in charge—your nurse and the technician—that it is important for your partner to have you with her. If you are not permitted to stay, ask the labor nurse who accompanied you to give your partner her support. Remind your partner that you will be right outside.

    You will have a short wait before you return to the labor department, to make sure all the pictures developed properly. If any did not, these will be re-shot.

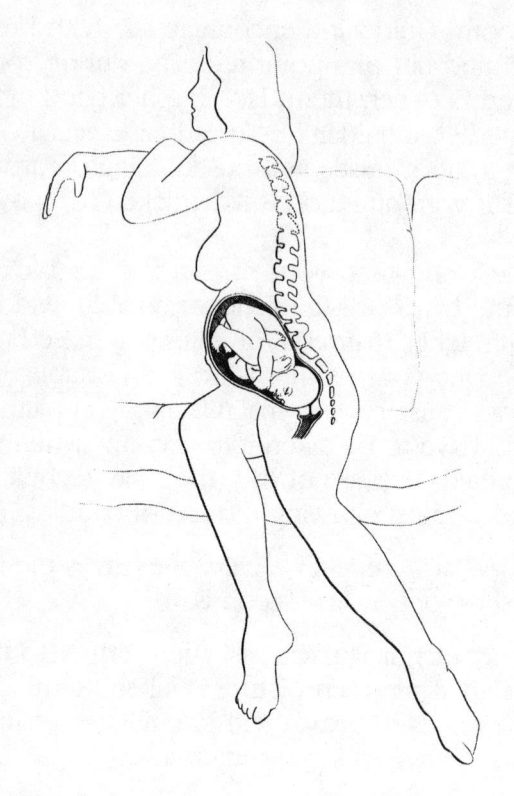

In back labor, baby's back is against mother's spine.

BACK LABOR

One out of 5 mothers has back labor, so named because the mother feels her contractions mainly in her back rather than in her abdomen. Usually, in back labor, the baby's back is against the mother's spine instead of her abdominal wall. This causes strong pressure against the mother's back. Because the pressure is from the baby's position, it lasts during intervals as well as during contractions (when the pressure is even stronger).

This pressure is hard to endure. It is painful, and there are no real rest periods, as there are with other labors.

Because of the way the baby's head lies against it, the cervix dilates slowly. Contractions are usually long, and come in an irregular pattern throughout the labor. The lack of a dependable rhythm makes breathing and relaxing more challenging. In this situation, labor tends to last longer than the average time.

As a coach, you will feel frustrated because you cannot change the situation. It is hard to see someone you love in pain.

- Inwardly, try to balance your concern with the decision to accept the situation. Decide that you will concentrate on offering all the support you can.

Most babies have to be in an anterior (back forward) position to fit through the pelvis at birth. Sooner or later, most back-labor babies do turn around. If the forces of nature do not turn the baby, forceps may be used during the delivery. For details, read about forceps on page 238. In certain positions, gravity adds a helpful influence.

To help the baby to turn around, suggest to your partner that she change her position.

- When she lies on her back, the baby rests against it.

- When she lies on her side, however, the baby rests forward, against her abdominal wall. Pillows behind her back, between her knees, and in front of her supporting her upper arm will make her more comfortable.

- She may want to be on her hands and knees (with the side rails of the hospital bed raised), so that the baby falls forward, away from her back. If she finds this position tiring, she can try kneeling in bed, resting her body forward against the raised hospital bed mattress with a pillow against her chest for comfort.

- She can kneel on the floor, resting her head and arms on a chair or couch.
- She can sit on a bed tailor fashion, with her body leaning forward and her head and arms resting on pillows in front of her.
- Sitting on a chair or the toilet, she can spread her knees apart and lean forward so that her belly rests between her thighs. You might sit in a chair in front of her, or put a table in front of her with a pillow on top so that she can rest her upper body there.
- Sometimes she will feel best standing up and leaning against you, or leaning over a table.

Unless your partner senses intuitively which position works best, she may need to try a few before settling on one. Some women try everything, and then prefer a semi-reclining position after all.

- Moving can seem impossible in the presence of back pain. Don't hesitate to ask a nurse to help you to encourage and assist your partner to change.

Counter-pressure can help to make back pain bearable. In most of these positions you can easily push with your hand against your partner's back.

- You and your partner will need to work together to find the exact place where pressure feels best. Between contractions, ask her to show you the right spot(s). It is usually somewhere above the division of her buttocks.

- Try a steady pressure, or a rotating pressure in which you make small circles with the heel of your hand, moving her flesh around against her backbone without sliding your hand over her skin (which can cause chafing).
- You will need to find out how much pressure to use. Mothers often prefer intense pressure and you may be surprised at how strongly your partner might ask you to push. To start, try firm rather than intense pressure. Between contractions, ask whether you are pressing hard enough. Your partner may have a bruise or two the next day, but you cannot hurt her or the baby. If you are worried about this, check with the nurse, midwife, or doctor.
- Occasionally, intense pressure causes more pain than it relieves. Every so often, ask for feedback.
- To keep from getting tired, place your elbow against your hip, then your hand against her back. Lean into the push with your body. Using your body spares your arm muscles.
- Safeguard your own back. Instead of leaning over as you push, place yourself so that you are pushing straight ahead. Kneel down, or raise the entire hospital bed to your hip level.
- If your partner is lying on her side, you may have to hold her in place with one hand on her hip as you push with the other hand. A pillow placed in front of her may supply extra support.
- If your partner is in a semi-reclining position, applying back pressure is awkward but still possible. She can lie on tightly rolled towels, sheets, or cotton blankets (wool blankets are usually too soft). She

can try tennis balls or rolling pins, though they may prove to be uncomfortably firm. She can lean against her fists, or against yours. Or you can place your hands, palms up, under her lower back and press or pull upward during contractions.

Heat or cold against the back can relieve pain. Heat relaxes muscles, cold numbs nerve endings.

- It is easiest to use 2 washcloths or small towels with a basin filled with very hot water, or very cold water (add ice chips). Wring one towel out well, and place it on the trouble spot on her back. Soak the other towel well in the meantime, to get it as hot (or as cold) as possible. Then wring it out and switch towels. Keep going this way.

- If your partner has no preference, try hot compresses during a few contractions, then cold compresses during a few. Ask her which feels best. Note: You can apply counter-pressure directly against the compress while it is in place on her back.

- You can also use chemical ice packs, wrapped in wet towels. These are cans or plastic bottles filled with a chemical that, once frozen, takes longer to thaw than water does. Get them from a grocery or hardware store well before the due date and keep them in the freezer. Remember to take them with you to the hospital.

- Many pharmacies sell another kind of cold, or hot, pack for first aid use. These stay cold or hot only 20 minutes or so, but are soft and flexible.

- Another trick is to half-fill 1 or 2 rubber examination gloves with cold water and ice chips for use as an ice pack, tying them off as you would balloons. You can ask the nurse to help you assemble them.

- Hot water bottles can feel good, but the temperature should be checked by a medical attendant to prevent burns. Most likely, you would need to bring a hot water bottle from home.

- Between contractions, ask her if she wants the compresses continuously, or just during contractions, or just during breaks. Trial and error will show both of you what works best.

With all of this for you to think about, your coaching tasks are still the same: timing contractions, checking breathing, and reminding your partner of 4-point releasing. Back labor is hard work. Your partner easily may become discouraged and tired. Your encouragement is especially important.

Nourishment supplies energy.

- Especially if your partner does not have an IV, you can offer sips of water, clear juice, tea with honey, unsalted or lightly salted broth, or an occasional spoonful of honey between contractions. Check first with your doctor or midwife to make sure your partner has permission to drink liquids.

As a coach, your effort will be constant. Short breaks can clear your head and renew your energy. Please read the section on helping yourself in Chapter 6, *Coach's Skills,* on page 101.

- Ask the nurse to fill in for you occasionally, whether or not you leave the room. This allows you to devote those few minutes fully to yourself. If the nurse is busy and cannot come at once, ask her when she can, and pace yourself accordingly. If time goes by and you wonder if she has forgotten, speak to her again.

- Tell your partner what you are going to do, why, and when you plan to be back. She can cope better if she knows exactly what to expect.

INDUCING AND SUPPLEMENTING LABOR

Inducing labor means that labor contractions are begun artificially, using a synthetic hormone called *pitocin*. Pitocin resembles a hormone called *oxytocin* that is made by a woman's body. Oxytocin helps to cause contractions of the uterus during labor. It works with several other factors in the mother's body to start off labor and to keep it going. Because several factors start labor, pitocin alone will not do it unless the uterus is ready.

Pitocin is given by IV. For more details, read about medications during labor on page 221.

Reasons for inducing labor:

1. When the bag of water breaks before contractions have started on their own, doctors often induce labor. The water bag bars the bacteria normally found in the vagina from entering the uterus. After the bag breaks, bacteria then may find a way in. While it is unlikely that they would cause an infection, it is possible. The longer the wait until the baby is born, the greater the likelihood of infection. Some doctors wait several days before inducing labor to see whether it will start on its own. The mother may be asked to enter the hospital where she can be checked often for any signs of infection.

Some doctors wait approximately 12 hours, while others induce labor right away.

2. When a mother has a medical condition that could cause problems for the baby in the last month of pregnancy (for example, diabetes, or Rh blood problems), labor may be induced when the baby is ready to live outside the uterus.

3. If a pregnancy lasts longer than 3 weeks after a due date that is known to be accurate, the placenta, now past its prime, can become less capable of nourishing the baby properly. Tests can show whether this is happening. If it is, labor may be induced.

> **Inducing labor for convenience, rather than for medical reasons, is not recommended.**

Reason for supplementing labor:
During labor, pitocin may be given to strengthen contractions if the midwife or doctor does not think the contractions are effective enough to move labor along at a reasonable rate.

Generally speaking, once a labor that starts spontaneously reaches the active labor stage, some progress is expected every hour. *On the average*, the cervix dilates about 1 centimeter every hour with a first-time mother, or about 2 centimeters every hour with other mothers.

A gentle labor that is progressing slowly but steadily, with mother and baby in good shape, will reach its goal without stimulation, and is easier for the mother to handle. Walking about, relaxing her mind and body, using breathing when necessary, and adequate rest and nourishment all encourage productive labor.

When the mother is in upright positions (standing, sitting, kneeling, squatting), gravity helps to bring down a baby that has not yet dropped fully into the pelvis. This in turn can bring about more effective contractions.

A uterus that has slowed down because it is tired often responds with renewed energy after the mother eats a spoonful of honey.

Coping with induced or supplemented labor:
Contractions induced by pitocin differ from those that start of their own accord. Mothers find that pitocin contractions peak quickly with little or no gradual build-up, are longer than average, and have shorter intervals. (Spontaneous contractions strengthen more slowly and follow a gentler overall pattern.) A pitocin labor almost always takes a few hours less than a spontaneous labor because the contractions are more powerful.

Pitocin contractions require steady hard work from your partner and you. You may find it useful to handle induced or supplemented labor as you would transition, using the ideas on pages 138 to 145 and in Chapter 9: *Coping with Pain,* on page 187.

Once pitocin has been started, it can be stopped at any time. A solution without medication added is run through the IV, or the IV is stopped altogether.

CESAREAN BIRTH

Some expectant mothers and fathers learn during pregnancy that their baby will be born via a Cesarean section. With this advance notice they have time to digest the news and to find out what to expect.

Most Cesareans, however, are the result of an unexpected turn of events during labor. For these couples, a Cesarean is an abrupt plunge into the unknown.

The idea of major surgery is frightening. During pregnancy, although you are likely to know that Cesareans happen, usually you have no reason to think your partner's labor may end in one. You prefer and are planning for a vaginal birth—so the idea is put from your mind. As a result, if that vague possibility suddenly becomes a reality, you may be shocked and not prepared to deal with it.

For you, the coach, the outlook changes dramatically. How can you help your partner now? Will you be in the way? How will the experience affect you?

By all means prepare for a vaginal birth. In addition, read and remember this section. Knowing some facts in advance—about Cesareans, the routines hospitals follow when one is performed, and what would be helpful for you as coach to know, before, during, and after an unexpected (emergency) Cesarean—will better equip you and your partner to change gears in midstream if you must. Having a baby by Cesarean is safer than ever before. Techniques and anesthesia are more refined, simpler, and quicker.

Reasons for planning a Cesarean:

1. You may know ahead of time that the baby cannot fit through the mother's pelvis. This may be because the baby is too big for an average-size pelvis, or because the pelvis is too small, or is unusually shaped for an average-size baby.

2. Sometimes the baby's position makes descent through the pelvis impossible—if, for example, he

lies across the opening instead of head first or bottom first.

3. In certain cases of toxemia, heart, or kidney disease, or with chronic high blood pressure, the hard work of labor would be too much of a strain for the mother.

4. Sometimes the placenta, normally located high up in the uterus, lies across the cervix or so close to it that it will separate as the cervix opens during labor. This cuts off oxygen to the baby and causes hemorrhage for the mother. It is called a *placenta previa*.

5. A mother with herpes simplex virus II may have active lesions in her vagina. These could infect the baby passing through the vagina.

6. The expression "once a Cesarean, always a Cesarean," is true only part of the time. A previous Cesarean may necessitate a second one, *if* the original reason for it still exists (a small pelvis or a chronic illness, for example), or possibly if a vertical (classic) cut rather than a bikini (low flap) cut was made in the uterus. You cannot tell this by looking at the abdominal scar because the cut on the abdomen may be different from the one in the uterus. The uterine cut should be noted in the records held by the doctor who did the first Cesarean.

Reasons for surprise (emergency) Cesareans:
The word "emergency" covers *all* Cesareans that are not arranged in advance. It does not always mean a true emergency, although it can.

1. Even though all signs during pregnancy may have suggested that baby and pelvis would fit each

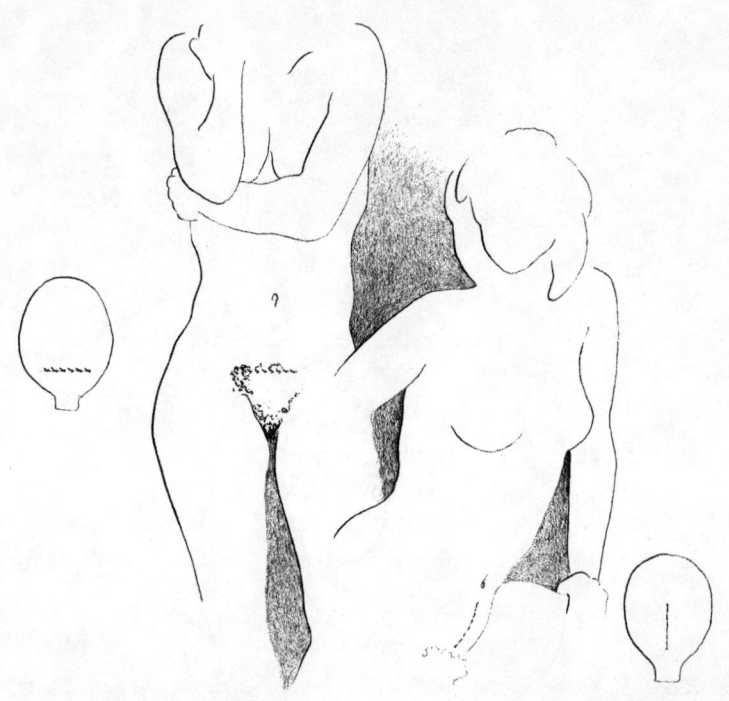

Bikini Cesarean incision   *Classic Cesarean incision*

other, it may turn out not to be so. When a period of labor with strong contractions has passed without the expected changes in the cervix, or without the baby settling down into the pelvis, the doctor may suspect a problem with measurements or position. To find out, he probably will order an x-ray (*pelvimetry*) of the mother's pelvis and the baby. This picture will show details of the baby's position and the size of baby and pelvis, so that he can tell whether a Cesarean is necessary. X-rays should be avoided during pregnancy, but are relatively safe now that the baby is fully formed.

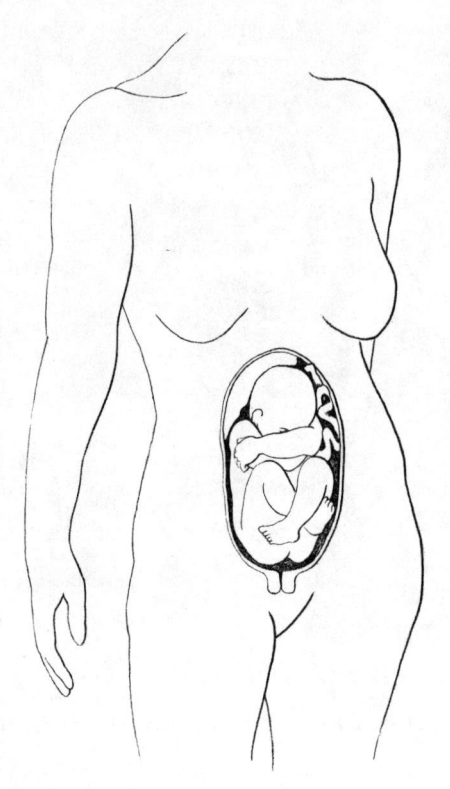

Baby in a breech position.

2. Because the birth is trickier if the baby is in a breech position, many doctors now deliver breech babies by Cesarean, especially if it is a first baby. Others turn to Cesareans only after a trial labor. Until recently, most breech babies were born vaginally.
3. After the bag of water breaks, there is a chance that infection may enter the uterus. If 24 hours pass without labor bringing the baby close to birth, the doctor may choose to deliver by Cesarean.

4. *Dystocia* means "difficult labor." It is due to any number of causes connected with mother and/or baby—ineffective contractions, a cervix that is unusually tight, an unusually shaped pelvis, a baby that is unusually large or in an unusual position, for examples. Often these difficulties can be remedied during labor and the baby can be born vaginally. If not, a Cesarean is the solution.

5. If the placenta separates from the uterus during labor, the mother loses blood and the baby loses oxygen. When a mother has periods of heavy bleeding during pregnancy, it is a warning that this condition may exist. The doctor will suspect that the placenta is likely to separate during labor, and make stand-by arrangements for a Cesarean. This is called *abruption of the placenta*.

6. Occasionally the placenta can separate during labor without advance warning. This would be a real emergency.

7. Contractions that stop or weaken, in spite of efforts to energize the uterus by releasing tension, walking about, using upright positions, rest, nourishment, or medication may make a Cesarean necessary. This is called *uterine inertia*.

8. Extreme changes in the baby's heart rate, beyond the normal range of 120 to 160 beats per minute during labor, may mean that a Cesarean is needed. To see whether these changes are temporary or continuous, the doctor is likely to use the fetal monitor (for details, read about the fetal monitor on page 213). The mother might be asked to breathe oxygen through a mask so that her blood carries more oxygen to her baby. If she lies on her

left side, freshly oxygenated blood is helped by gravity to flow more quickly through her body. Often, the baby's heart-rate changes are due to pressure on the cord, which slows the supply of oxygen to the baby. This is called *fetal distress* and is a true emergency.

9. If the cord drops below the baby and is compressed between the baby and the pelvis as the baby moves down, oxygen to the baby is cut off. Until the Cesarean is done, the mother's bed is tilted head-down to use gravity to keep the baby's head away from the cord. Often a medical attendant helps to hold the head back with her fingers in the vagina. This is another true emergency. It is called a *prolapsed cord*.

What to expect with a Cesarean:
As soon as you know a Cesarean is possible, and especially when the doctor decides to do it, both you and your partner may experience a variety of feelings. Each of you might feel tremendously relieved that a long and difficult labor will soon be over. At the same time, each of you may be very disappointed that the birth will not be the way you had hoped. It might relieve you both to shed some tears. You both may be scared, wondering if everything will be all right. If you are asked to leave the labor room, loneliness may increase your fears, and your partner's as well.

Your room suddenly may be filled with people and action. As the staff moves quickly, preparing your partner, they may have little time to explain things—especially if the situation is a true emergency.

The best way you can help is to give your attention to your partner. She will appreciate your personal support while the staff is busy with procedures and paper work.

- Encourage her to carry on with relaxation and breathing. Contractions will continue, and so will the need to cope with them. She is still in labor and must work with her contractions until she is given anesthesia, after she reaches the operating room. It is hard to keep going without the vaginal birth as a goal. On top of this, both of you are experiencing strong emotions. Sticking with the methods of support you practiced together for so many weeks will help both of you to remain calm.

- Relaxing is especially important now, for you as well as for your partner. Remember that letting go of physical tension helps you to stay on top of things when you feel nervous. As you guide your partner through releasing, let go of your own tension, point by point. Talk quietly but firmly. Touch her gently.

- Find out if she has questions you can ask for her. Though the staff is busy, they will answer questions whenever they can. Watch for an opening. If you are unsure, you could start by saying "May I ask a question?"

- If you see small ways that you can help the staff, by all means offer, as long as it does not take you away from your partner when she needs you.

- In a true emergency you may be asked to leave immediately. *Before* labor begins, ask the doctor or midwife *and* the nurse in your hospital's labor and delivery department if coaches are allowed to stay in the labor room during preparations for a Cesarean.

Preparations for a Cesarean:
Preparations for a Cesarean delivery include several steps. Each takes only a few minutes. For more details on some of the procedures, read the fuller descriptions of each in Chapter 11.

A **consent form** is signed by the mother, giving the doctor permission to do the Cesarean. If she is medicated, her husband or legal guardian may sign. If she is not yet of legal age and not emancipated (that is, if she is not yet legally responsible for herself), her legal guardian may sign. Procedures vary from one locality to another.

A medical attendant **shaves** the mother's abdomen, her pubic hair, and sometimes the top of her thighs.

An **IV** is started, if one is not already running.

One end of a **urinary catheter** (a long skinny tube of plastic or rubber) is put into the mother's bladder through her urethra (the opening to her bladder, located just above her vagina). The other end of the catheter attaches to a plastic bag that is hung at the side of the bed. The bladder, empty of urine, will remain out of the way during surgery.

- As the catheter is put into the urethra, your partner may feel temporary pain or pressure (as though she needs to urinate). Guide her with 4-point releasing and whichever breathing helps the most.

Blood may be drawn from a vein in the mother's arm by a technician from the hospital laboratory. Even though blood may have been drawn when the mother was admitted to the labor room earlier, extra blood tests usually are needed for surgery.

Medications may be given to the mother, usually

by mouth or by injection, to help her relax, dry her mouth, and/or settle her stomach.

The anesthetist who gives anesthesia for the operation may visit now to ask the mother a few questions —whether she has recently had anything to eat or drink, whether she is allergic to any medications—and to explain the kinds of anesthesia he plans to use. (Also read about anesthetics on page 221). He will answer questions too, as long as he has time. Sometimes he waits to talk to the mother after she arrives in the operating room.

Your partner will be brought to the operating room in her bed or on a stretcher. Either of these can fit in the elevator if surgery is on another floor. Usually coaches may go along as far as the door to the surgery department. Unless there is a need to hurry, the staff will wait if you ask, while you give your partner a hug and a word of encouragement.

- You can tell your partner that you will be thinking of her, and that you will be waiting to see her and the baby. If she will not be awake for the birth (as she would be with spinal anesthesia), she may be reassured to know that you will be seeing the baby about 10 or 15 minutes after the birth. Even if this is a true emergency and there is little time, a kiss, a hug, a squeeze of her hand can express what may be hard for you to say.

During the surgery, you might wait in a waiting room just outside the surgery department or back in the fathers' waiting room on the maternity floor, depending on how this is handled in your hospital. Waiting can be difficult. You may feel isolated, worried, and if a lot of time passes, forgotten. You may find yourself wondering if the Cesarean happened because you weren't good enough at coaching—even though you know, reasonably, that it happened for reasons beyond your control.

- If it helps, find a nurse—or a medical attendant to tell you where one is—and ask her the questions you have on your mind. There is usually a pay telephone near the waiting room. Calling to talk with a person close to you might help to ease your worries.

A Cesarean birth takes about 1½ hours. The baby is born within 5 to 15 minutes. Most of the remaining time is needed for stitching the uterus and the muscles and skin that cover it (the abdominal wall).

Afterward, the mother goes to a recovery room for 1 to 3 hours. There, a nurse watches her very closely, checking on her blood pressure, pulse, and breathing, and making sure her incision and uterus are all right. After the anesthesia wears off and all her systems are working normally, your partner will move to her room on the maternity floor.

Unless it is the hospital's policy to keep mother and baby together, the baby is brought from the operating room to the nursery very soon after being born. Whether you are waiting outside the surgery or in the maternity waiting room, be on the lookout for the baby. Usually you may walk to the nursery with the baby, who is transported in a roll-along warmed crib.

- Ask if you may watch inside the nursery or through a window, while the nurses weigh and measure the baby, take footprints, put on identification bracelets, and give eyedrops and a shot of Vitamin K.

- Someone might invite you to put on a gown and go into the nursery to hold the baby. If not, do not hesitate to ask if you may. Holding the baby will be a moment you will always treasure. Also, it will be an experience you can describe to your partner when you see her.

- Remember all the details you can, especially the baby's weight, length, and facial features, to tell your partner.

Depending on the hospital's policies and on the doctor, you may be able to visit your partner in the recovery room.

- While you wait, find out from a nurse if this is possible, and ask her to call you when your partner has returned from surgery and you may go in.

- If you go to the recovery room, you will want to know what to expect. The nurse caring for your partner can answer most of your questions. Specific details about your partner or the baby will come from the doctor. For more about the recovery room, see page 270.

In the operating room:
Your hospital may be one that invites fathers into the operating room for the Cesarean birth of their babies. If you are not the father, you may be able to go along as coach. Many hospitals require a certificate showing that you took a class on Cesareans, or at least that you have written permission from the obstetrician. At least a month before the due date, prepare for this possibility.

You may never have thought that you would want to be present for surgery. But it may surprise you to realize that, after hours of working together in labor, you do not want to be separated. Continuing to be together is reassuring to your partner as well as to yourself. And you may want very much to be present when the baby is born.

- If you think of it as you leave the labor room, bring along Chapstick and a wet washcloth to soothe her lips or to cool her face.

Even if you are already dressed for the delivery room, you will be given a change of clothes after you and your partner enter the surgery department. These are the "scrub" clothes worn by nurses and doctors. While you change, your partner will be wheeled into the operating room.

- You may feel better about leaving your partner alone if you ask a nurse to help her with relaxing and breathing during the few minutes you are apart.

After you have changed, wash your hands so you can touch the baby after birth. You will have a short wait outside the operating room itself while your partner receives her epidural, or spinal. If she is to have a general anesthesia, which is given a few seconds before the actual operation starts, you may be able to go in as soon as you are ready. Please read about medications on page 221.

- In any case, be sure to get permission from a medical attendant before you enter the operating room. You will be given a cap, face mask, and covers to wear over your shoes. You must put these on before you go in. (More details are on page 151.)

Operating rooms look just the way you might expect they would: they have tiled walls, a few stainless steel stools and tables, and green, blue, or white sheets draped over everything. They often lack windows. You will see a long table with a great variety of instruments for this operation, in all shapes and sizes. At the head of the operating table, where you and the anesthetist have seats, will be an impressive-looking machine composed of tanks, tubes, and dials. This contains oxygen and other gases. There is also a machine to monitor blood pressure. Near the operating table you may see a suction machine that removes fluids, such as water from the amniotic sac, while the Cesarean is going on.

By now your partner will be on the operating table and you can take a seat by her head. In order not to touch anything as you walk through the room, it is easiest if you keep your arms at your sides, folded across your chest, or behind you with your hands clasped.

A vertical screen is placed over your partner's shoulders so that neither of you can see the surgery when it is going on. You may touch your partner anywhere on your side of the screen.

- Your partner may find it tremendously reassuring if you talk with her quietly or simply hold her hand. The smallest gestures can bring great comfort.

- If you brought Chapstick and a wet washcloth, now may be the time to use them. Check with your partner and also with the anesthetist if he is nearby.

- To steady yourself, check inwardly for tension and let it go with 4-point releasing.

- Continue to help your partner with relaxing, as well as with her breathing. Remember that she will keep on feeling contractions until she has anesthesia, when they will continue without her awareness until the baby is born.

Because your partner has an IV in one arm and a blood pressure cuff on the other, each arm rests on a board attached to either side of the operating table. As preparations for the Cesarean birth continue, a nurse washes your partner's abdomen with an antiseptic solution the color of iodine.

With spinal anesthesia or an epidural, your partner will not feel her body from her chest down.

- She needs reassurance that this is normal and that the numbness will wear off within a few hours.

Because breathing muscles work differently with spinal anesthesia, your partner may have the sensation that she is not getting enough air. She also may feel nauseated.

- Speak to the anesthetist sitting beside you. He might give her a whiff of oxygen to relieve these discomforts.

If your partner is not numbed by spinal anesthesia, she may feel cold because operating rooms usually are cool.

- You can ask a nurse to cover her with blankets or sheets.

The anesthetist can also answer questions and pass on requests. Although he is busy, he usually has spare moments. If you should feel lightheaded or nauseated or unwell in any way, he (or a nurse, if one is nearby) is the person you should tell. In such a situation it is best to speak up and take steps to help yourself rather than simply wishing the symptoms would go away.

Some of the doctors and nurses in the room have had the same experience at some time during their training.

- Talk yourself through 4-point releasing and at the same time take very slow long breaths in through your nose, blowing them out through pursed lips.

- Don't hesitate to put your head down between your knees. Someone might break an ammonia capsule under your nose.

- If you would like to leave the room, say so and someone will walk you out.

- Outside, feel free to sit right down on the floor if a chair is not in sight. Give yourself credit for having the courage to take care of yourself. If it is permitted, you may want to return when you feel better.

Two doctors, one of them your partner's obstetrician, and a nurse work together to perform the Cesarean. A second nurse runs errands and fetches things. A pediatrician may be in the room to check the baby immediately after birth.

After the surgery begins, the **baby will be born** within 5 to 15 minutes. Your partner may feel some tugging when the baby is lifted from her body.

The first step is to **suction the baby's nose and mouth** and to stimulate breathing, just as it would be for a vaginal birth. Cesarean babies sometimes need extra suction because they miss going through the vagina, which squeezes out excess lung fluids.

Next, **the cord is cut**.

Before the doctor places the baby in the warmed crib that has been brought into the operating room, he may hold this marvelous tiny child above the screen for you and your partner to see. If the baby is not held up, imagine the frustration for a mother when everyone can see her baby except herself, positioned as she is behind the screen. In your excitement you may forget this.

- Describe everything you can see about the baby. If your partner has questions, be sure to answer them, even if you have to say "I don't know" or "I can't see." She will feel less helpless if she can count on you to hear her and act as her eyes.

You may feel torn between going over to the crib to look at the baby and staying with your partner.

- Ask her how she feels about it.
- Be sure to ask a doctor or nurse if it is all right to move around to the crib. Get permission before you touch anything, even the baby. The wonder of birth makes it hard to remember that this is an operating room.

Usually, after the initial examination the baby is wrapped warmly in a blanket, carried over to be shown to your partner, and perhaps given to you to hold.

- If this doesn't seem to be happening, you can ask the anesthetist or a nearby nurse if it could be arranged.

- If your partner's arms are restrained, you or the nurse can lay the baby's face against hers. This skin-to-skin contact is very important because it will give her a bit of the closeness she had looked forward to with a vaginal birth. If the anesthetist feels it is safe, he may remove the blood pressure cuff temporarily so that your partner can have one arm free to hug and touch her baby.

At this point, some women feel tired and dazed from all that has gone on. Your partner might have difficulty concentrating on the baby and prefer to wait until later to become acquainted.

After a few minutes the **baby may be taken to the nursery** on the maternity floor of the hospital.

- You can ask your partner if she would prefer that you go to the nursery with the baby (if hospital policy permits) or remain with her.

Some hospitals keep parents and baby together without separation after a Cesarean, if there are no complications. Some bring the baby to the recovery room after the mother arrives there.

- If your hospital has no provision for mother and baby to be together during recovery, perhaps your doctor can arrange it if you discuss it *ahead* of time, and remind him when surgery is over. The more time Cesarean parents—particularly the mother—can spend with their baby, the quicker they will recover from the emotional shock and loss caused by the surgical, instead of vaginal, birth.

After the placenta has been removed by hand from the uterus, your partner's **incision will be repaired,** taking about 45 minutes. Your partner may feel drowsy now and doze off and on. Sometimes gas is given for a short sleep.

Later, your partner will go to the recovery room, and then to her room. If she had wanted rooming-in, the baby may remain in the nursery except for feedings until your partner feels up to changing and lifting the baby herself. If fathers, usually the only visitors allowed in the rooming-in room, can spend a few hours helping with baby care, the baby may room-in earlier.

In the recovery room:
Every patient responds differently during the first hours after surgery. If your partner had general anesthesia, she may feel groggy, dizzy, or nauseated. After an epidural she may remain numb for up to 3 hours. After a spinal she may be numb for up to 6 hours and will be asked to lie flat for up to 12 hours.

Once the anesthesia has worn off, your partner may have medication for pain. If she plans to breastfeed, the doctor can suggest the medications that will have the least effect on the baby. Pain comes from the incision and from contractions as the uterus tightens and becomes smaller, something it would have done during birth if your partner had had a vaginal delivery.

- You can remind your partner that the pain is usually strongest right after surgery, and will let up noticeably day by day.

- If your partner's mouth is dry and she is not awake enough to swallow fluids, you or the nurse can help her to rinse her mouth or to wet her lips with water. Vaseline or Chapstick feels wonderful on dry lips.

To clear her lungs of mucus, your partner will be asked by the nurse to breathe deeply, cough, and turn from side to side. She may be afraid to do this because it hurts.

- Gentle encouragement can help a lot. Coughing and breathing are easier if your partner does it while pressing her hands or a pillow directly against the bandage over her incision.

- Between these efforts, you can remind her of 4-point releasing and slow breathing.

Your partner may have many questions about the baby, only a few, or none. If she was asleep for the birth, she may find it difficult to believe that the baby has been born until she feels her flattened abdomen with her hand.

- Tell her all the details about the baby you can think of.
- Some hospitals will bring a healthy newborn into the recovery room for the mother to see and hold. Ask if this is possible. It is the best way for her to know she is really a mother, and to feel close to her baby.
- She may feel weak and shaky. If so, you can help her to hold the baby. Placing the baby on her chest near her face (away from her tender abdomen) may give her the closest contact. Unwrap a little hand or uncover the baby's cheek for your partner to touch. The baby's soft skin feels more real than a blanket-wrapped bundle. If you feel unsure of yourself, ask the nurse for suggestions.

If your partner feels up to it, she can try breastfeeding. Her least uncomfortable positions will be to lie flat or slightly raised with the baby lying across her chest, or to roll onto her side with the baby beside her.

- The baby might turn out to be sleepy, or not interested. Remind her that not all babies are eager to nurse at first, and a little while after birth most babies take a nap.

The baby may not be with your partner during this recovery period.

- When she is ready to go to her room, ask the nurse if you can all stop by the nursery. Ask the nursery nurse if she could bring the baby out to your partner so that they can greet and touch one another. This is a contact that touches the heart, and it is immensely important for mothers. More than having had surgery, she has just given birth.

Afterward:
In her room at last, your partner's incision, vaginal discharge, and her vital signs (blood pressure, pulse, and breathing) will be checked by a nurse. It is very likely that she will feel like sleeping, though pain and excitement may make it difficult. A comfortable position with lots of pillows for support, pain medication if she needs it, and a reminder from you about head-to-toe releasing can help a lot.

A word on the **pros and cons of using medication for pain:** Pain causes tension and fatigue. When it is reduced—or absent—the body's energy is freed from the task of fighting pain and can be used for healing. Sleep and rest become possible. This helps a new breastfeeding mother to manufacture milk.

Knowing that most medications pass through her milk to her baby, a Cesarean mother may consider taking none for the pain. Before making such a decision, she will want to look at how medications affect the baby (the effects vary; some are slight), how uncomfortable she is, and how else she can lessen pain by relaxation, changing position, mild exercise, and hot water bottles.

People are rightly cautious about routinely popping pills, and they wisely seek alternatives. Medications have their merits, too, and may be the best choice at times. Decisions will be based on the balance of pros and cons for each individual.

- Suggest that your partner talk with her obstetrician and pediatrician about medication and the baby. La Leche League (an international information service for breastfeeding families) has a complete list of drugs and their effects on babies when received through breast milk. The telephone numbers of members near you may be obtained from the obstetrician, pediatrician, hospital nursery, other nursing mothers, or white pages of the phonebook, listed under La Leche League.

After your partner is in her room, you may want to sit quietly together for a little while.

- Before you leave, ask her whether you can do anything for her, or bring her anything the next time you come to visit.
- Tell your partner where you will be after you leave, when you will call if she has a telephone by her bed (some hospitals have only telephone booths for patient calls), and when you will return.
- Tell the nurses where you can be reached. Ask when you may visit and, if the baby has brothers and sisters, whether they may visit, too.

You may want to hold off most other visitors during the first week or two, in the hospital and at home, to give your partner a chance to rest and to get to know the baby.

After you leave, you may feel greatly let-down that the birth was so different from what you and your partner worked so hard for, especially if you wound up in the waiting room and missed it altogether. You also may feel relieved and happy, and probably tired. If there are sisters and brothers who are waiting for the news of the baby's birth, you will

want to take the time to give them enough details to
satisfy their interest. You may want to share your experience
with some people close to you before you
get some sleep. Treat yourself in some special way.
Most people will ask about your partner, not realizing
that you have had your own intense experience.
Bravo and congratulations to you, too!

> **Help** with cooking, shopping, and housework is
> essential for at least 2 weeks. Your partner is recovering
> from surgery as well as from labor, and
> she is undergoing physical changes from a pregnant
> to a non-pregnant state. She needs rest and
> mild exercise, and should use her energy to enjoy
> and care for the baby and for the physical
> changes taking place within her, not for household
> chores.

For the next few days:
For your partner, walking and showers usually start
within 1 or 2 days after surgery. The catheter usually
is removed within 6 to 12 hours, the IV within 1 or 2
days. Meals will start with clear liquids and go on to
foods that are easy to digest and then to a regular diet.

After abdominal surgery the intestines are slow to
pass gas out of the body and foods that cause it, like
broccoli, cabbage, and beans, should be avoided. Moving
about, especially walking, as early as possible is a
big help in stimulating the intestines to function normally.
It also encourages good circulation and brings
about faster healing. Sitting still makes the body stiffen
up so that pain gets worse.

Stitches (or clips, or staples) are removed on day
5 to 7. Mothers often go home on the same day or
soon after.

13. Loss

During pregnancy, most parents imagine many things about the coming baby—appearance, personality, sex, and what life will be like together. This imagined baby is a kind of dream baby who will be replaced by the real baby when he, or she, is born.

Parents also wonder and worry about whether the baby will be healthy. These concerns are hard to talk about and, especially because the outcome can't be known until birth, usually are unresolved and tucked quietly away. Although most of the time these fears turn out to be groundless, occasionally they are not. A small number of babies may be born with a problem, or stillborn.

For parents, this is a time of shock and sorrow. Not only have they lost the baby of their dreams—a loss common to all parents—but the adjustment to so unexpected a reality is far more difficult than they may be prepared to handle.

Each such situation is unique, but many of the reactions and resolutions are shared by those who also have been through the experience. These guidelines touch briefly on feelings, suggestions, and information. Further help can come from medical people, clergy, therapists, books, organizations, and parent support groups geared to these special situations. Ask your hospital, doctor, and childbirth teacher for names. Please also see *Further Reading,* on page 299.

A PREMATURE BABY

A baby is classified as premature when she weighs under 5½ pounds at birth. No longer is the date of her arrival compared with the date she was due—due dates are too undependable. The obvious characteristics of these little newborns are their skinny appearances, reddish and transparent-looking skin, and labored breathing. Because the life force is wonderfully powerful, most of these babies come through the first days—or weeks—of special care as fit as any other baby.

A baby weighing more than 5½ pounds and yet showing signs of being physically immature may also need special care until she grows stronger and adjusts to life outside the uterus.

When labor starts too early, the doctor may try to stop it by giving the mother certain medications, including alcohol, intravenously. Should labor continue anyway, it will be not much different from any other labor except that it may move along more quickly. The smaller baby slips into the world more easily.

It is the mother who needs constant emotional support, plus constant physical guidance. Knowing that her baby may have a problem, she is worried and scared. She should never be alone unless she specifically says she wishes to be. And then someone should always be within easy calling distance.

A baby in trouble at birth is taken immediately to the nursery. Although special care begins right away, usually some time must pass before the doctors can predict the baby's future definitely. The uncertainty is trying for parents. Sometimes medical attendants hesitate to talk openly, concerned about upsetting them. Facts are easier to cope with than the unknown.

- Ask as many questions as you need to ask.
- Make your wishes about being given information very clear to the doctors and nurses in charge.

It is very important that parents and baby spend time together, no matter how brief, as soon as possible after the birth. This creates a bond with the baby and helps to fill the empty spaces in the mother's and father's hearts. If a transfer to a large medical center is being arranged, the meeting is even more important.

- Try to spend time together with the baby every day. Many hospitals provide low-cost rooms in the hospital or in homes nearby, for parents who live far away.
- If this is impossible, try to get a snapshot of the baby.
- Visits and daily phone calls to the hospital nursery can help parents to feel connected with their baby.

Though parents very much want to touch their baby, they often are afraid of disturbing something. The doctors and nurses, who touch the baby as they care for her, can show you what you need to know.

- Diapering the baby, feeding her (breast milk is the best food for a baby with problems), caressing her, and calling her by name all help her parents to realize that she is truly theirs, not the hospital's.

Contact of any sort helps to make the baby seem less of a stranger, more a part of her family, when she comes home at last. Approximately one-third of all abused children begin life as premature babies, who were separated at birth from their parents for long periods of time so that the parent/baby relationship did not have a chance to form.

A LESS-THAN-PERFECT BABY

More than 96 percent of births are normal. But occasionally a baby is born with a birth defect or injury. The problem may be correctable with surgery—sometimes immediately, sometimes at a later date. Some situations are beyond the powers of medical knowledge, and will become a permanent part of the lives of these parents and their child.

If the newborn with a birth defect or injury is taken immediately to the nursery, or if a mother is asleep for the birth, her coach may know before she does that there is a problem. Untruths and evasions can cause more concern than simply-told facts. This must be made clear to medical attendants in charge, who sometimes sidestep the truth to protect parents.

When a coach is uncertain about what to say, intuition can be a good guide. Usually it is a dependable source of sound advice, especially as the coach probably knows the mother better than anyone in the hospital. Also, a coach can turn to midwife or doctor, and compassionate staff members, and talk over questions with them.

As soon as possible after the birth, both parents should participate in taking care of their baby. Separation, particularly in these circumstances, interferes with attachment between parents and child. For mothers especially, feelings are two-sided—a yearning to nurture and care for the baby that conflicts with a natural impulse to turn away from her. Parents need to learn to relate to a child who was not a part of their dreams during pregnancy—to a stranger, in a sense. They are now faced with the reality that their child will require much care and attention, perhaps always.

Often parents have mixed feelings about being with their baby in the hospital. They are frightened, and not sure how they will react to the obvious physical problems as well as the hospital machines and routines. Yet they find that, when they are with their baby, they gain tremendous emotional satisfaction from relating to her as a whole child, a person, instead of thinking about her from a distance, as a collection of problems.

Accurate information on the nature of the problem is vital to these parents. Their own midwife, doctors, and hospital nurses can explain many things. They also can refer them to specialists and organizations covering the area in question, parents in the same situation, and books. Suggestions also may come from their childbirth instructor, La Leche League, or instructors of obstetrics or pediatrics at nearby schools of nursing or medicine.

Because so much is unfamiliar, support and guidance from professionals is essential. From family and friends, this mother and father need reassurance about their own adequacy as parents. They will benefit from understanding that their own feelings, though perhaps unexpected and even disturbing, are normal under such circumstances.

THE LOSS OF A BABY

A baby who dies during pregnancy, at birth, or shortly afterward, is real to his parents, however short his life. Yet because death is a hard subject to face, loved ones, friends, even medical attendants, not knowing what to say, often say nothing or push the subject aside, or negate its importance, talking around it. Sometimes people try to erase the pain by erasing the event—"It is for the best" and "There can always be another"—treating death as a bad dream best forgotten.

Yet this baby's few months of life have affected his parents and changed them. He already holds a place in their hearts. His loss through death is real.

Death must be faced to be dealt with. Parents report that seeing and touching their child helps them to accept the loss. Possibly other loved ones may wish to see and hold the baby. Being together makes the baby real as a person, and gives the family someone to whom they can say goodbye. Compassionate doctors and nurses can arrange a time to be with the baby and offer support as it is needed.

Because the shock is so great at first, it may be difficult for parents to think clearly. Arrangements may leave out things important to them—baptism, taking a photograph, saving a lock of hair. Practical arrangements are particularly difficult if parents are under pressure to make immediate decisions. If some decisions—such as working out funeral arrangements—can wait a few days, parents have the chance to consider their own wishes and to think a little more clearly.

Understandably, coaches wonder how they will react to so unexpected and difficult an event as illness, birth defects, or stillbirth. Couples who have been together during such an experience say that the presence of the other gave each of them comfort and support that would have been missing had they been apart and alone. Having someone known and caring nearby lessened fear and strengthened courage. It was easier to remain calm when it was important to be so.

- At the time of birth, and later during your partner's hospital stay, sharing your feelings together may be the greatest help you can offer.

- When she leaves the hospital, you can recognize that for her it is uniquely painful to be without the baby who had been a constant part of her until now.

- You can also help by acting as her liaison with the professionals who will be part of your lives for awhile. Your partner will have questions that need answers, requests that need responses. You yourself may find additional help through sharing your experiences and feelings with compassionate listeners, especially people who have been through the same experience.

GRIEVING

The array of feelings that confront grieving parents can be overwhelming. Whether the cause is death or change, as with an ill or handicapped child, grief has many levels that usually move through us in a predictable order, often overlapping.

At first it is normal **to feel numb**, constantly or on and off for minutes, days, or weeks. The facts are hard to believe.

As the truth becomes real to us, it is normal **to become angry**. The anger stems from a feeling of helplessness. We ask the question, "Why me?"

It is normal also **to blame ourselves** for what has happened and to feel that we are being punished. As we try to find a cause, we list things that we (or another) might have done differently. At this point it is important to know all the facts surrounding the problem. Usually they were beyond the parents' control. Even if they were not, they must be faced and accepted for future peace of mind.

In addition, it is normal **to feel guilty** about our grief and its demands on others. Not only do we have the right to grieve, but it is essential for our emotional health that we do so.

Depression, another part of grieving, may be emotional—we feel sad, confused, listless, worthless, and so involved with sorrow that our hearts seem empty of love for people dear to us. Depression may also be physical—constipation, headaches, loss of appetite, trouble with sleeping. Thinking clearly may be difficult, and it is common to act impulsively when making decisions. When the decisions are important, take the time to make them carefully.

Fear is also part of grieving. To be afraid that another hurtful thing may happen to others we love, or to ourselves directly, is a normal protective reaction, not a forecast. Children, especially, feel and express this fear.

Eventually, we can begin **to face reality**. Our pain is released. We may express it through intense weeping or talking or both. While our sorrow becomes more bearable with time, acceptance cannot be rushed. Recovery time varies from person to person. The loss never goes away, and there will be periods of intense sadness. Patience is a most important help, taking the task one day at a time. After awhile, the future starts to look brighter, and we begin to feel that we can plan for it.

For the parents of of a handicapped child, grief cannot be resolved completely because coping with the problem becomes a part of their lives. Assistance and support are especially important so that they can find room for happiness, satisfaction, and productivity.

TELLING OTHER CHILDREN IN THE FAMILY

When parents have other children, telling them what has happened can be less difficult than it might seem. Holding back information confuses and scares children; it does not protect them. Sharing feelings with them is realistic because they know, at any age, that their parents are acting differently from the way they usually act.

Honesty works best. Children sense it when parents sidestep the truth, and they wonder and worry about what is hidden. Explanations should be short and simple. Young children have difficulty understanding abstract concepts like God and heaven. They understand what they see and feel.

Children grieve too, and they need to express themselves for the same reasons their parents do. They may need to be encouraged to bring their feelings out into the open. Often, children express themselves by behaving, or asking questions, in unexpected ways at unexpected times. Some ponder in silence and, in an effort to maintain their own inner balance, they may seem to go on with life, untouched.

All children need reassurance that they are safe from the problems the baby had; that their family, which is clearly in turmoil, is not falling apart; that they are still loved. At times, when parents are using all their energy to meet their own needs, it may be difficult or impossible to meet the needs of their children. It can help to call on other loving people to offer comfort and support to the children at these times.

COPING WITH LOSS

In coping with their loss, parents need:

1. To be able to support each other and communicate with each other;
2. To be able to explore their own feelings;
3. To be able to say what is on their minds;
4. To be able to ask questions and to receive answers.

Grief must be expressed to bring relief. Locking away feelings means that they are held inside us forever. If we suppress them until a more convenient time, it is harder to let them out.

The relationship between parents can be weakened by grief. A father, not knowing how to handle his sorrow, or feeling that it is unmanly to express it, may avoid the issue by keeping to himself, perhaps away from home. A mother, feeling that she is imposing, may not reach out for the support she needs. Parents need to listen to each other. It is important to talk, even if words seem inadequate at times.

Sometimes silence brings the greatest relief. Sometimes the intensity of grieving can be eased by sharing with other people—relatives, friends, medical people, counselors. Some people, including family, seem insensitive because, not knowing what to say, they often say nothing or even stay away. Some seem to expect life—and us—to go on as normal, as though nothing at all has happened. But when we express ourselves, we are more likely to receive the support we are looking for. Often, people simply are waiting tactfully for us to speak first; some can help better after we explain our needs.

Talking with other parents in the same situation can help to bring feelings to the surface, to understand and release them. Sharing similar experiences brings comfort and support.

It is best to wait until the grieving has run its course before starting another pregnancy. No child can be replaced by another, and parents must find a place in their hearts for this one, before another follows. Please see *Further Reading* on page 299 for books and organizations that may help in coping with loss.

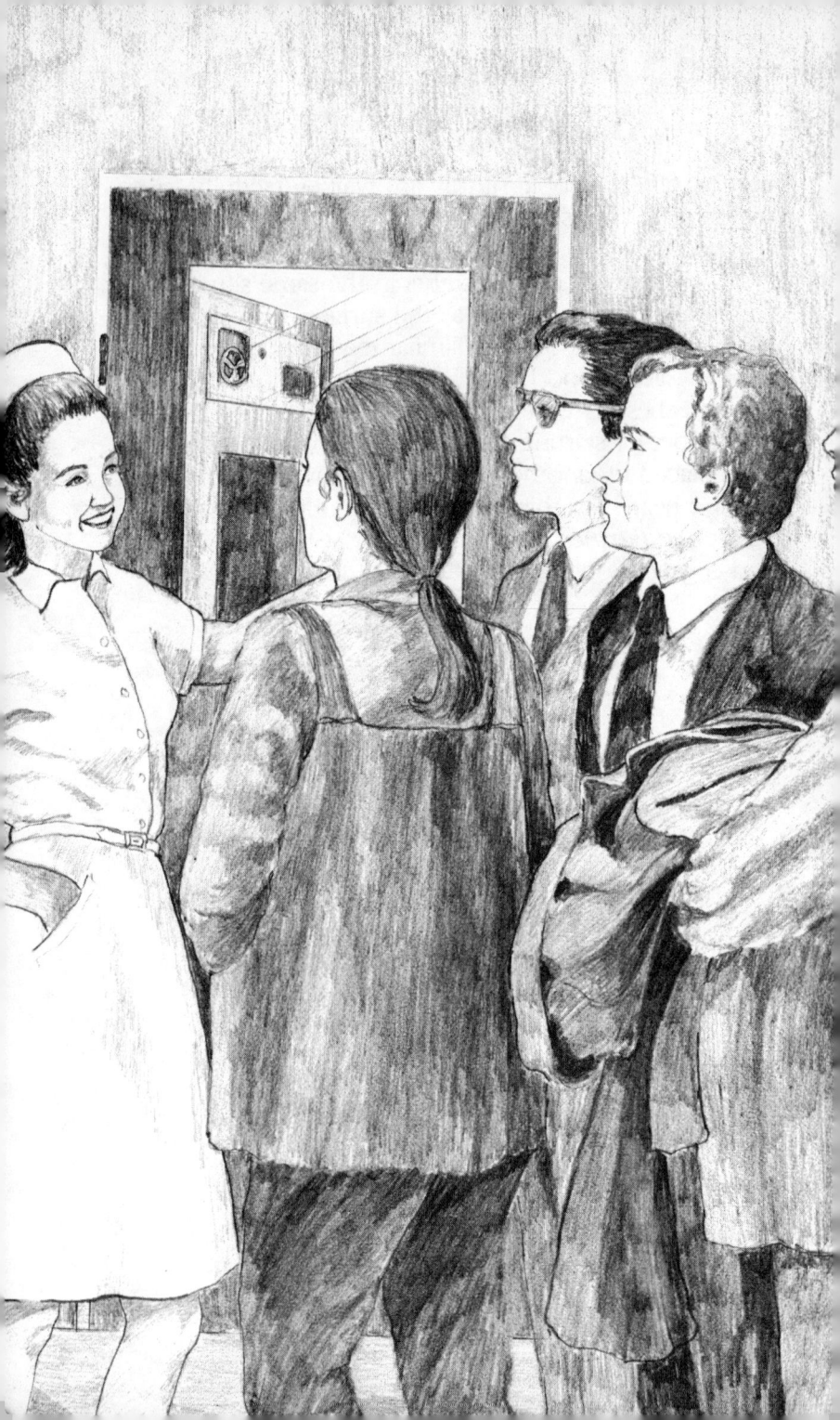

14. Lists

Planning for labor and birth is at least part of ensuring a satisfying experience—and for any planning, lists are helpful. Here are three: questions to ask the hospital staff, questions to ask your midwife or doctor, and things to bring with you when you go to the hospital.

QUESTIONS TO ASK THE HOSPITAL IN ADVANCE

Get to know your midwife or doctor and your hospital *before* labor begins. If you know the answers to all the following questions, you will have a good idea of what to expect from your environment during labor and birth. You may learn a lot of these facts during office visits, childbirth classes, and the hospital tour, without having to ask. Use the list of questions below as a guide to fill in the gaps in your knowledge.

Hospital facts:

1. Does the hospital have a school of nursing, midwifery, or medicine?

    Will student nurses, midwives, interns, residents be taking part in our labor (asking questions, performing procedures and vaginal exams)?

    Is the midwife or doctor willing to go out of her or his way to do these procedures personally or to request a staff nurse to do them, if your partner prefers it this way?

2. Are there midwives on the staff of the hospital?

   What is their function?

3. Does the hospital have an early-labor lounge for mothers and coaches in early (warm-up) labor?

4. Does the hospital have a birthing room?

   What are the procedures for its use?

   Are there special circumstances when your partner would not be allowed to use the birthing room?

   Where would she labor instead?

   Where would she deliver?

5. Does the hospital have a birthing chair?

   A delivery table with an adjustable back rest?

6. Does the hospital have rooming in?

7. What is the hospital's Cesarean rate?

8. Is an anesthetist on call for obstetrics in the hospital 24 hours a day?

9. Where do coaches wait if they are separated from their partners during labor? During delivery? During recovery? During a Cesarean?

   Is there a fathers' waiting room?

10. Where may coaches change their clothes?

11. Where is the coach's bathroom?

12. Where in the labor room are these items: Basins? Hot and cold water? Ice chips? Warmed blankets? Extra linen?

Matters usually decided by hospital policy:

13. Does the hospital permit coaches to be with mothers during labor?

14. Does the hospital permit coaches to be someone other than the husband—for example, an unmarried father? Relative? Friend?

15. Are mothers and coaches separated at any time during labor, birth, or afterward? For example:

    If the couple has not taken, or not finished, childbirth classes?

    During the mother's admission to the labor room?

    During hospital procedures (enemas, IVs, shaves, lab technician visits, vaginal exams)?

    During midwife or doctor visits?

    When medications are given in labor?

    For birth?

    In the delivery room?

    In the recovery room?

16. What is the step-by-step admission procedure in the hospital?

    May any forms be filled out in advance?

    Does your midwife or doctor add or subtract any steps?

17. May mothers keep personal belongings (i.e., eyeglasses, jewelry) during labor? Birth? Cesareans?

18. What do coaches wear in the labor room? For delivery? For a Cesarean?

    Will they put on masks, caps, and paper shoes?

19. May mothers bring and use extra pillows from home?

    Should they supply their own pillow cases?

20. Can coaches expect help with coaching from staff members?

21. How soon after birth may a mother hold her baby? Breastfeed? Drink and eat? Get up? Telephone her family? See her family? When may the coach hold the baby?

22. How long do mother, coach, and baby stay together after the birth?

    If they are separated, how long before they can be together again?

23. May photographs be taken during labor? Delivery? Afterward?

    Are flash attachments allowed, as long as the flash is not directed at the baby's eyes?

24. May coaches come into the operating room for a Cesarean?

    Are only fathers admitted, or any coach chosen by the mother?

    For the coach to be present, is it necessary to show a certificate from a class on Cesareans?

    Is it necessary to have written permission from your doctor?

25. May coaches accompany the baby into the nursery after a birth?

After a Cesarean?

26. When the mother has rooming-in, who may visit?

May baby and visitors be together in the same room?

27. May Cesarean mothers room in with their babies?

Can they room in sooner if the father, or another companion, stays in the room to help with the baby?

28. In rooms for mothers who do not have rooming-in, may fathers stay for feedings?

May other visitors?

29. Are babies brought to mothers on a 4-hour schedule or when they are hungry (a demand schedule)?

30. What are hospital procedures for a baby who is premature? Ill? Stillborn?

Are parents included in the procedures?

May they see and care for their baby?

31. May brothers and sisters of the baby visit the mother during labor? Birth? Immediately afterward?

Is there an age limit for children visitors?

May they touch and hold the baby?

QUESTIONS FOR MIDWIFE OR DOCTOR

32. When in labor is your partner asked to come to the hospital by the midwife or doctor?

May she spend early (warm-up) labor at home?

33. Does your midwife or doctor permit mothers to eat or drink after labor begins?

34. If you have a midwife, who is the doctor who is her backup?

How do his policies compare with hers?

35. If your doctor is not available, who stands in for him or her?

How closely do the policies of the substitute compare with those of your doctor?

36. If your partner's water bag breaks while she is still at home, when should she come to the hospital?

37. May mothers remain out of bed for labor?

38. When will your midwife or doctor join you at the hospital?

39. If your doctor or midwife is not yet at the hospital and a staff member refuses you permission for something your midwife or doctor agreed to let you do, is it all right with her or him if you ask that she or he be telephoned for confirmation?

Is she or he willing to give you written permission to take to the hospital when labor starts?

40. Under what circumstances does your midwife or doctor use pitocin? Rupture the membranes? Use the fetal monitor? Start an IV?

41. What kinds of medications does your midwife or doctor use for labor? For birth? For a Cesarean?

Under what circumstances does she or he offer these?

42. What is your doctor's Cesarean rate?

Under what circumstances does he believe that Cesareans are necessary?

43. If your partner has a Cesarean, who will perform the operation?

Who assists this doctor in performing a Cesarean?

44. How does your midwife or doctor feel about using the birthing room? A birthing chair?

How does she or he feel about mothers' giving birth in the labor room bed?

About using pillows on a delivery table that is without a back rest?

45. What people might be in the delivery room, in addition to the mother and coach, midwife or doctor, and 1 or 2 nurses?

Will a resident midwife or doctor assist with the birth?

Will your midwife or doctor support your wishes if you prefer only the minimum number of people?

46. May your partner use the position of her choice for the birth?

Does your midwife or doctor prefer a specific position?

47. When using a delivery table, may your partner avoid using the stirrups if she feels more comfortable without them?

48. Under what circumstances does your midwife or doctor perform an episiotomy?

Will she, or he, use active support (perineal massage, hot compresses, stirrups close together or no stirrups, gentle pushing) to avoid an episiotomy when possible?

49. During delivery, are restraints placed on the mother's arms? On her legs?

Are sterile drapes used?

50. Is it possible to have dim lights, quiet, and a warm bath for the baby at the time of delivery?

May the coach give the bath?

51. What are your doctor's or midwife's policies on suctioning the baby? Cutting the cord?

52. May your partner hold the baby skin-to-skin, wrapped in a warmed blanket, immediately after birth?

When may the coach hold the baby?

53. Are eye medications for the baby routinely used at birth?

May the parents have permission to delay these for 1-2 hours, in order to make eye contact with the baby?

54. How does your midwife or doctor feel about circumcision?

How soon after birth does she, or he, perform a circumcision?

Do other doctors substitute?

55. If you, the coach, need to leave the delivery or birthing room at any time, are you permitted to return? When?

If you leave the operating room during a Cesarean, may you return?

ITEMS TO BRING FROM HOME FOR LABOR

Note: You may use everything on this list, or only one item, or nothing. You can't know in advance, so bring it all just in case. Be prepared.

1. **Your partner's insurance card**.
2. **A letter or a certificate** as proof that you and your partner took classes in childbirth education. If information on Cesareans was also taught, this should be mentioned.
3. **This book**, for reference if you need reminders.
4. **Your special request list**, covering your special wishes for labor and birth.
5. **Pen or pencil, and a pad of paper**, to keep track of the pattern of contractions as well as for questions and requests that you both want to remember.
6. **Watch, with a second hand, or stop watch**, for timing contractions.
7. **A focal point**, a picture, flower, little toy or item of the baby's clothing, something special that your

partner can gaze at while concentrating during contractions.

8. **Long, warm socks.** Laboring women can have cold feet in labor, even in summer.

9. **Chapstick, Vaseline, cream** for keeping your partner's lips moist.

10. **Lemon wedges or sour candies** to keep your partner's mouth moist if she is not allowed to drink liquids once labor starts. Lollipops can be put aside easily when a contraction begins.

11. **Mouthwash**, for rinsing after long periods without taking fluids, or after throwing up—or for you, if your partner is extra sensitive to food smells or cigarette smells.

12. **2 washclothes**, home-washed with no hospital detergents to taste if a cloth, dipped in cold water, is used to wet your partner's dry mouth. A wet cold cloth is also used for back compresses or a refreshing wipe-down, over her face especially, when she is hot and tired.

13. **Cornstarch or unperfumed powder** in a shaker can for massage, stroking, and back rub.

14. **Hot water bottle and ice pack** for back labor compresses.

15. **Small (5 x 10½ inch) paper bag** for your partner to breathe into (if she prefers it to cupped hands) to stop signs of hyperventilation.

16. **Extra pillows** inside plastic bags or pillow covers, labeled with your partner's name on adhesive or masking tape.

17. **Food**.

For you:

Hearty bean or meat soups in a thermos.

Meat or peanut butter sandwiches on whole wheat bread.

Cheese, wrapped to keep it fresh.

Raw fruits and vegetables.

Mints or gum.

For your partner, if she is allowed nourishment by mouth:

Clear liquids such as homemade non-salty broths, tea with honey, cranberry, apple or grape juices. These can be frozen in ice cube trays and broken into chips. Bring liquids to the hospital in thermos bottles.

Easy-to-digest foods for after labor, such as homemade non-salty soups with pureed or well-cooked vegetables, homecooked (no additives) cornstarch puddings in plastic containers, crackers.

Note: Check with your midwife or doctor to make sure that your partner has permission to eat these, or other foods, during labor.

For you both:

A bottle of champagne for after-birth celebration.

18. **Time passers**: books, magazines, diary, card or board games, small portable TV for early or slow labor spent in the hospital.

19. **Camera and film**: Use high-speed film (ASA 400) if you will not be using a flash.
20. **Nickels, dimes, and quarters** for telephone calls, soda vending machines.
21. **List of people to call after the baby arrives.**

15. Further Reading

CHILDBIRTH CLASSES

Hotchner, Tracy: *Pregnancy and Childbirth*. Avon Books, New York, 1979. An encyclopedic 689 pages packed with information on all aspects of pregnancy and birth. Very thorough, straightforward, clear, and supportive of parents.

PREGNANCY AND BIRTH

Bing, Elisabeth: *Six Practical Lessons for an Easier Childbirth*. Grosset & Dunlap, New York, 1967.

Ewy, Donna and Roger: *Preparation for Childbirth*. New American Library, New York, 1970.

These both are excellent textbooks describing the traditional Lamaze method of preparation for childbirth.

BORN ON THE WAY TO THE HOSPITAL

White, Gregory J., M.D.: *Emergency Childbirth*. Interstate Printers and Publishers, 1958. Available from the Police Training Foundation, 3412 Ruby St., Franklin Park, Ill, 60131. A 64-page manual of facts and directions for the emergency birth attendant. Simply and clearly written.

CIRCUMCISION

Wallerstein, Edward: *The Circumcision Decision*. 1980. The Pennypress, 1100 23rd Avenue East, Seattle, Wash., 98112. A pamphlet explanation of the history of circumcision, its development through today, with medical and public opinion. Taken from Edward Wallerstein's book *Circumcision: An American Health Fallacy*.

MEDICATION AND DRUGS

Adrian, Betsy K., and Nada Logan Stotland, M.D.: *The Medication Chart*. 1981. Available from ASPO, 1411 K Street NW, Suite 200, Washington, DC, 20005. A large, single-page chart written in academic style, bearing complete information on most of the drugs used during labor, birth, and Cesareans. Listed are 51 reference sources used by the authors.

CESAREANS

Donovan, Bonnie: *The Cesarean Birth Experience*. Beacon Press, Boston, 1977. Information from A to Z on Cesareans for parents and professionals.

PREMATURITY

Hospitals with nurseries that are equipped to care for premature babies usually print information booklets for parents, explaining equipment and procedures.

BIRTH DEFECTS AND BIRTH INJURIES

Roberts, Nancy: *Help for the Parents of a Handi-*

capped Child. Concordia Publishers, St. Louis, Ill., 1981. Educational and practical information written with understanding and concern.

GRIEF

Miles, Margaret: *The Grief of Parents When a Child Dies*. 1978. Compassionate Friends Headquarter, PO Box 1347, Oak Brook, Ill., 60521 (Telephone: 312-323-5010). A compassionate, informative booklet that will help grieving parents to understand and cope with their sorrow. The organization, The Compassionate Friends, offers guidance and information to grieving parents, including help with finding or organizing parent support groups.

16. Glossary

A

Active labor: The phase of labor's Stage 1 that comes after early labor and before transition. See pages 14 and 133.

Admissions procedures: The steps taken to admit a mother to the hospital or birthing center. For details, see page 205.

Advanced breathing: Labor breathing skill with a complex pattern and rhythm to match especially demanding contractions. Also called *Emergency Breathing*. See page 35.

Afterbirth: The placenta, cord, and amniotic sac expelled during labor's Stage 3, after the baby's birth. See page 172.

Amniotic fluid: Water inside the amniotic sac that surrounds the baby before birth. See page 72.

Amniotic sac: The thin-walled sac inside the uterus, surrounding the baby and containing amniotic fluid.

Analgesic: Medication that relieves pain. See page 225.

Anesthesia: Medication that causes loss of feeling or consciousness. See *Medicines and Drugs* on page 224.

Anus: Opening between the buttocks into the rectum.

Apgar Score: A method for judging the baby's condition within a few minutes after birth. See page 177.

B

Back labor: Type of labor that occurs when the unborn baby is positioned with his or her back facing the mother's spine. See page 244.

Bag of water: Another name for the amniotic sac.

Birthing center: Place, often independent of a hospital, where a mother may labor and give birth in a setting as homelike as possible, in the company of loved ones.

Birthing chair: A chair with a U-shaped seat on which a mother may sit to give birth to her baby. See pages 49, 55.

Birthing room: A private room, located within a hospital's labor and delivery department, where a mother may labor and give birth as naturally as possible, with a minimum of interference and a maximum of support for her body's functions.

Birthing stool: A U-shaped stool to support a mother as she squats to give birth. See page 53 for details on positions.

Bloody show: Bloody, mucous vaginal discharge from the dilating cervix at the beginning of, and during, labor. See page 72.

Bradley method: See *Lamaze method*.

Braxton-Hicks contractions: Mild contractions of the uterus that take place throughout pregnancy. See page 76.

Breaking of the waters: Breaking of the amniotic sac.

Breathing skills: Skills learned by the mother to help her to work with labor contractions. See pages 29 to 43.

Breech: The baby's position in the uterus when the buttocks, knees, or feet are the part of the baby that will pass first through the cervix.

C

Caput: Small section of the baby's head that appears at the outer opening of the mother's vagina shortly before birth. See page 149.

Catheter, urinary: Thin tube passed into the bladder to empty out urine.

Centimeter: Measurement equal to about half an inch, used to figure out how far the cervix is dilating in late pregnancy and during labor. Ten centimeters is full dilation. For details on stages of dilation, see page 14.

Cervix: Opening at the bottom of the uterus like the neck on a turtleneck sweater. See page 12.

Cesarean: Birth of a baby through an incision made in the mother's abdomen and uterus. See page 252.

Chux: Absorbent pads placed under a mother during labor to catch fluids from her vagina.

Circumcision: Cutting away the foreskin from the boy baby's penis. See page 220.

Cleansing breath: Deep, slow breath taken to announce the beginning and ending of a contraction. See page 23.

Clear fluids: Semi-transparent liquids that do not contain fat or food particles. For example, tea, ginger ale, apple juice, water, broth. See page 81.

Coaching clothes: Special clothes that hospital policy might require a coach to wear in the labor, birthing, or delivery room. See pages 91 and 151.

Combination breathing: Using two or more breathing skills for a single contraction, changing from one to the other to match the changing strength of the contraction. See page 34.

Concentration: One of the essential labor skills, the ability to center one's attention without being diverted by distractions. See page 22.

Contractions: Tightening of groups of muscles of the uterus that will eventually bring a baby to birth. See page 76.

Control: In labor, control means the ability to work with, instead of against, one's body during contractions.

Crowning: The appearance of a large area of the baby's head at the vaginal opening, with bulging of the mother's tissues.

D

Delivery, or birth: The moment the baby leaves the mother's body and enters the world. See *Chapter 7*, page 127.

Delivery table: A table with a mattress, sometimes an adjustable back, and stirrups, on which a mother may give birth.

Demonstration: One of the coach's tools, the acting out of a particular labor skill for the mother's benefit. See page 112.

Dilation: Opening of the cervix that begins in the last 6 weeks of pregnancy and is completed during labor, measured in centimeters or fingers.

Drugs: Any substance that, when taken into the body, will change some part of its function. See page 221.

Dystocia: A difficult labor with specific causes centering around mother or baby.

E

Early labor: Beginning of labor, with warm-up contractions that are mild and bring about only slight progress. See pages 14, 76, and 127.

Effacement: Flattening of the cervix, beginning during the last 6 weeks of pregnancy and completed during labor.

Effleurage: Light stroking of the mother's abdomen.

Emergency breathing: Labor breathing skill with a complex pattern and rhythm to match an especially demanding contraction. Also called *Advanced breathing*. See page 35.

Emesis basin: Small, kidney-shaped basin that is used to throw up into.

Encouragement: An important part of a coach's help to a mother in labor, using words to strengthen her resolve to work with her labor, and her belief that she can. See page 103.

Engagement: The point of labor at which the baby's presenting part (usually the head) has settled down into the mother's pelvis.

Epidural anesthesia: Injection of anesthesia between two vertebrae (back bones) low on the back, outside the spinal cord. See page 228.

Episiotomy: Incision, or cut, of the perineum shortly before birth. See page 217.

F

Fetal distress: Extreme changes in the unborn baby's heart rate caused by conditions that are overly stressful for the baby.

Fetal monitor: Machine used to record the baby's heartbeats, and the length and strength of labor contractions. See page 213.

Fetoscope: Special stethoscope designed to pick up the sounds of the unborn baby's heart beating.

Fingers: Measurement used to figure out how much the cervix is dilating in late pregnancy and during labor. Five fingers measures full dilation. See also *Centimeters*.

Focal point: Anything at which a mother gazes to help her concentrate. See page 24.

Focus: One of the laboring woman's aids, the act of gazing at, or resting one's eyes on, a focal point to enhance concentration. See page 23.

Forceps: Skillfully designed tools to help a baby to be born. See page 238.

Foreskin: Skin covering the end of the penis. See page 220.

4-point releasing: Conscious, concentrated effort to let go of tension throughout the body by focusing on four specific body areas: face/neck/shoulders, hands, bottom (perineum) and thighs/feet. See page 27.

Fundus: The body of the uterus.

H

Hyperventilation: Imbalance of oxygen (too much) and carbon dioxide (too little) in a person's circulation. It can result from imbalanced labor breathings. See page 235.

I

Induced labor: Labor contractions that are started artificially, usually by giving the medication pitocin to the mother. See page 250.

Inertia or uterine inertia: The stopping or weakening of labor contractions in spite of steps taken to reenergize contractions. See page 257.

Internal exam: Vaginal exam given by the nurse, midwife, or doctor to find out how far labor has progressed and how much the cervix has effaced and dilated. See page 206.

Intervals: The rest periods between contractions.

IV or intravenous: A mechanism by which fluid, medication, or blood is given through a tube placed in a vein. See page 212.

L

Labor: Contractions of the uterus that efface and open the cervix and push the baby out into the world.

Labor room: Hospital room in which mothers and coaches spend the majority of labor, until delivery.

Labor skills: Relaxing, breathing, and pushing techniques used by the mother to work with her body during labor. See *Chapter 3: The Mother's Skills for Working with Labor*, beginning on page 21.

Lamaze Method: Both Lamaze and Bradley methods endorse parents' rights to be informed and involved consumers of their own medical care. Practioners of both offer courses for expectant parents, including facts on birth, pros and cons about medical techniques and hospital policies, and skills for mother and coach. Bradley places special emphasis on relaxing and slow, deep breathing. Lamaze, in addition to relaxing and slow, deep breathing, teaches shallow breathing techniques, and emphasizes precision and practice to create built-in responses to contractions.

Leboyer Method: Special attention given to the baby during birth and directly afterward, with dim lights, quiet voices, gentle handling and massage, and a bath. See page 219.

Losing control: See *Control*, above. See also *Chapter 9: Coping with Pain*, page 187.

M

Meconium: A baby's first bowel movement, dark olive-green in color. See page 73.

Medication: Drugs used for specific treatment. See page 221.

Membrane: Another name for the amniotic sac.

Midwife: A person specially trained to give medical care to a woman during her pregnancy, her labor and delivery, and the weeks immediately following the birth. A *lay midwife* learns her skills through experience. A *Certified Nurse-Midwife* (CNM) is a registered nurse with additional training at a school of midwifery, and certification according to the requirements of the American College of Nurse-Midwives. Some states require midwives to be licensed before they may practice in that state.

Mucus plug: Small mass of mucus within the cervix keeping bacteria out of the uterus during pregnancy. Passing the mucus plug results in *bloody show*, one of the signs of the beginning of labor. See page 71.

N

Nitrazine paper: Yellow test paper that turns blue when wet with amniotic fluid. See page 72.

No-push breathing: Emergency breathing used when the urge to push must be controlled. See page 35 and 51.

O

Observation: One of the means through which a coach helps to guide a mother in labor. See page 103.

Opening up: In labor, refers to a mother's conscious effort to release tension or to let go in her perineum as she pushes the baby out of her body. See page 45 and 146.

Oxytocin: Hormone made by a woman's body that causes contractions of the uterus. See page 250.

P

Pelvimetry: X-rays taken of mother's pelvis and unborn baby, to see the position of the baby as well as the size of the baby and the pelvis in relation to one another. See page 241.

Perineum: Small patch of muscular, elastic tissue located between the anus and the vagina.

Pitocin: Man-made hormone used to induce or to supplement labor contractions. See page 250.

Placenta: Round, flat organ that grows against the inner wall of the uterus. It transfers oxygen, nutrition, carbon dioxide, and waste products between baby and mother and is expelled from the mother's body as part of the afterbirth. See page 172.

Positions for birth: Positions that aid the descent and birth of the baby during the second stage of labor, and in which a mother feels comfortable. See page 53 and 152.

Positions for labor: Positions that encourage the uterus to contract efficiently and productively, and in which a mother feels comfortable. See page 135 to 138.

Postpartum: The period after the birth.

Praise: A coaching tool. Its purpose is to strengthen a laboring mother's self-confidence, by emphasizing her successes as she works and rests. See page 104.

Premature baby: A baby weighing less than 5½ pounds at birth, with other physical signs of prematurity. See page 276.

Presenting part: The part of the baby (usually head or buttocks) that will pass through the cervix and vagina first, during birth.

Progress: Changes in the cervix and downward movement of the baby caused by uterine contractions during labor and birth.

Prolapsed cord: Umbilical cord that has dropped beneath the unborn baby during labor and/or birth. See page 258.

Pushing urge: Desire felt by the laboring mother to bear down, usually at the end of the first stage or the beginning of the second stage.

R

Read Method: An approach to working with labor and birth that emphasizes education and relaxation as a way of overcoming pain.

Recovery room: The place where, after birth or surgery, a mother is closely watched for 1 to 2 hours, or as long as necessary.

Rectum: Last section of the intestine, 4 to 6 inches long, leading to the anus.

Regaining control: See *Control*, above. See also *Chapter 9. Coping with Pain*, page 187.

Relaxing: See *4-point releasing*, above.

Rupture of the membrane: The breaking of the amniotic sac. See page 72, 216.

S

Saddle Block: Injection of anesthesia between two vertebrae (back bones) into the spinal fluid surrounding the spinal cord. Causes numbness from the hips down. See page 229.

Scrub clothes: Special clothes worn by nurses, midwives, doctors, and coaches for Cesareans and usually for labor and birth as well. See pages 91 and 151.

Shallow breathing: Light, easy, short breaths used to work with labor contractions when they are too demanding to be matched by slow breathing. See page 32.

Silence: Often essential to enable a laboring woman to concentrate and work with her contractions. See page 109.

Silver nitrate: Medication frequently used to treat newborn babies' eyes as protection against eye infection caused by possible contact with gonorrhea germs in the mother's vagina. See page 219.

Slow breathing: Gentle, effortless, long breaths used before other breathings when breathing with contractions becomes necessary. See page 30.

Spinal anesthesia: Injection of anesthesia between two vertebrae (back bones) into the spinal fluid surrounding the spinal cord, causing numbness from the lower part of the ribs down. See page 230.

Stages of labor: Three divisions of labor and birth—effacement and dilation, birth of the baby, and passing of the afterbirth. See page 14; *Chapter 7,* page 127.

Staples: Used sometimes instead of stitches to close the skin after a Cesarean; removed before the mother leaves the hospital.

Stillbirth: A baby who is not living at birth. See *Chapter 13. Loss*, page 275.

Stirrups: Padded leg and foot supports that attach to a delivery table or birthing bed and that may be used by the mother while she gives birth.

Supplementing labor: Use of pitocin to strengthen contractions of the uterus during labor. See page 250.

T

Talking: Important coaching tool that provides communication between the mother and her helpers. See page 107.

Tired uterus: See *Inertia*, above.

Touching: Important coaching tool used especially for reminders to relax, and for communication and comfort, as well. See page 105.

Transition: Last of labor's three Stage 1 phases; brings strong contractions, a variety of emotional and physical changes, and the most rapid progress of this stage. See pages 15 and 138.

U

Umbilical cord: The cord that stretches between the baby's abdomen and the placenta during pregnancy.

Uterine inertia: See *Inertia*.

Uterus: A muscular bag containing the baby during pregnancy that, during labor, contracts and relaxes over a period of hours to pass the baby out of the mother's body.

V

Vagina: Canal leading from the mother's cervix to the outside of her body, just in front of her anus.

Vaginal discharge: During labor, the mucusy, bloody flow coming naturally from the dilating cervix. See page 72.

Vaginal exam: See *Internal exam*.

Vital signs: Blood pressure, pulse, and respiration—signs that can be quickly and easily checked to determine a mother's overall condition. See page 206.

W

Warm-up labor: See *Early labor*.

X

X-rays: A way of photographing bones and organs inside a living being. See page 241.